The Community is my University

A voice from the grass roots on rural health and development

Selina Maphorogo and *Erika Sutter*
edited by *Jennifer Jenkins*

Dedication

I want to dedicate the book to my husband and to my children,
because they were those who gave me permission to be away
from home to work with the community and to seek for new skills.
Secondly, to my co-workers who were working with me co-
operatively, for all the support they gave to me, and to all the
Care Groups who did all this beautiful work. I am also very
thankful to Dr Erika Sutter, who was not selfish in keeping her
knowledge for herself, but who was keen to share it with me.

Selina Maphorogo

Front cover: *details from a printed cloth for the 10th anniversary of the Care Groups by Palatsina Hlungwani, and printed by Tiakeni Textiles.*
The whole wall hanging is reproduced on page 6. It illustrates many of the varied activities of the Care Groups.
Back cover: *Selina Maphorogo and Erika Sutter discussing the book.*
(photo: M. Dörig)

© 2003 Royal Tropical Institute, Amsterdam

KIT Publishers
P.O. Box 95001
1090 HA Amsterdam
E-mail publishers@kit.nl
Website www.kit.nl/publishers

Graphic Design
Grafisch Ontwerpbureau Agaatsz BNO, Meppel, The Netherlands

Printing
Meester & De Jonge, Lochem, The Netherlands

ISBN 90 6832 722 4
NUR 130/890

Swiss Tropical Institute
Institut Tropical Suisse
Schweizerisches Tropeninstitut

Socinstrasse 57 Postfach
4002 Basel http://www.sti.ch/

KIT
PUBLISHERS

Contents

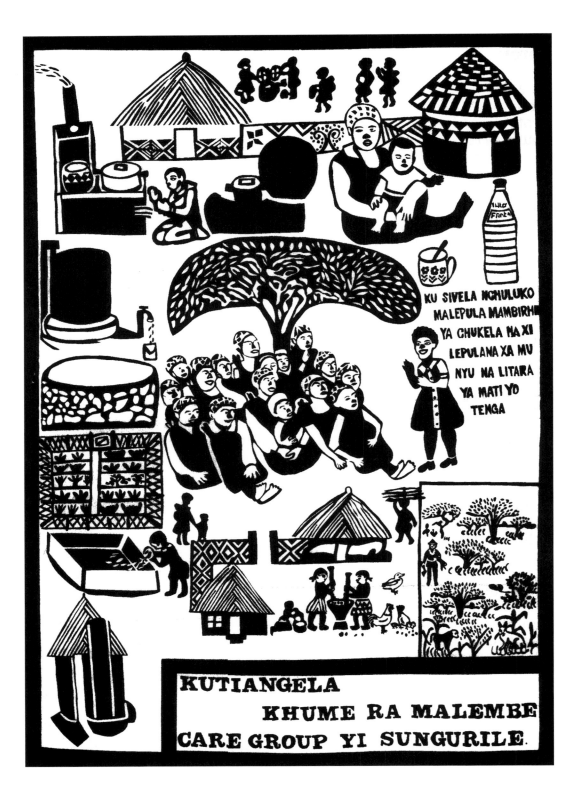

KU SIVELA NCHULUKO
MALEPULA MAMBIRHI
YA CHUKELA NA XI
LEPULANA XA MU
NYU NA LITARA
YA MATI YO
TENGA

KUTIANGELA
    KHUME RA MALEMBE
CARE GROUP YI SUNGURILE.

Foreword

Dr Mamphela Ramphele
Managing Director, World Bank (Health, Education, Social
Protection) formerly Vice-Chancellor, University of Cape Town,
South Africa

History is littered with narratives of people moving 'from rags to
riches'. There are fewer stories of those who have come from
poverty who not only succeeded in setting themselves up for
success, but also sought the path of success through enabling
others to succeed. Even fewer are cases of such path-breakers out
of the pit of poverty being celebrated by their own communities or
the wider society. This book embodies an extraordinary narrative
of a path-breaker with a difference. The narrative is a reflection
on the work of an extraordinary woman: rural in background; poor
in socio-economic terms; not highly educated by every account,
including her own; and courageous in every sense of the word.

To move from being a domestic worker to being a major player in
community health is no mean feat. To do so not only in one's own
village but to extend one's reach regionally, nationally and internationally is truly amazing.

The book is also a celebration of a powerful enabling partnership –
a partnership between an extraordinary missionary medical officer
and eye specialist in Tropical Health, and this poor rural woman.
Selina and Erika have over the last two decades become synonymous
with principled partnership. Theirs embodies the best there is in
such partnerships between bio-medical professionals and local
communities; women of different social classes; urban and rural
people; missionaries and those on the receiving side of their
ministry; North and South, and most importantly, human beings
inspired by the passion to do all they can to make the world a
better place.

The book also breaks new ground in documenting the experience
of the partnership – lessons learned and hopes for the future – by
the member least expected to do so. Too many poor, rural people
with a low level of education are frustrated by not being able to
reflect on their intellectual contributions to development, because

they lack the capacity to do so. There are many barriers to capturing one's narrative on paper: self-confidence, language (the dominance of English as the language of international discourse is a major constraint to those not educated enough to have scaled the fence), the commonly held view that writing is for specialists and not for ordinary people, and finally, time for reflection and writing – a difficult commitment to make in a rural environment where intellectual work is not necessarily seen as work. Selina has scaled all those barriers.

This book documents how careful, patient grass-roots work, if properly undertaken, can change the lives of rural communities in a sustainable way. Erika Sutter as an eye specialist recognised that she would not win the war against a common yet curable and preventable disease of the tropics, trachoma, unless she enlisted the support of the community she served. She recognised the importance of women in taking responsibility for the well-being of their families. She also recognised the power of knowledge in healing processes, and had confidence in the ability of uneducated people to grasp the logic of science and its methods if given the opportunity to do so. She enlisted and enabled women to use their positions of power to transform their own and other people's lives. The Care Group method of community empowerment in health care has been proven to be a cost-effective and efficient, sustainable method of enabling poor communities to take charge of their lives through sharing knowledge, and changing customs which are detrimental to health promotion and disease prevention. Many public and community health workers in South Africa have come to take this methodology for granted. It is however not an easy way out as Selina so eloquently documents. There are tears and sweat in the process of getting buy-in, motivating participants to stay the course, dealing with conflicts within and outside the group, and with individual members, going the distance when one is weary and frustrated etc. But it works.

This book should become recommended reading for those embarking on a career of empowering poor people wherever they are in this increasingly unequal globalising world. It gives one a window into the complexities of the empowering process. It also gives one hope. The scientific method is not only for the educated. All human beings given the opportunity to learn have the capacity to use science to solve the many problems confronting humanity.

The book is also fun to read. Too many of us have forgotten how far South Africa has come in the post-apartheid era. The divide between black and white South Africa was not just reflected in opportunities but in very basic things that middle class people take for granted. Selina records some of these: the difference between a 'big chicken' and a turkey; the experience of air travel for the first time when she went to visit Erika in Switzerland, and many other simple protocol issues which make human communication easy in homogeneous communities.

I am proud to have shared the Northern Province of South Africa as a birthplace with Selina. I was also privileged to have Erika as a supportive medical colleague and empathetic teacher in tropical health and hygiene during the dark years of banishment in the Northern Province. Even more wonderful is to have both women as my friends. I commend this book to all those interested in making a difference in our global village.

Acknowledgements

First and foremost we want to thank the people, both old and young, in the many villages in the north-eastern corner of South Africa, who shared their problems and their wisdom with us. From them we learned many things that helped us to shape the successful community project described in this book. We especially want to thank the thousands of Care Group members whose enthusiasm has sustained the Project for nearly thirty years. Their demands to know more, and to start new activities, motivated Selina to go on learning.

We are also grateful for the active support we received in various ways from people too numerous to be named individually. They include the members of the Top Executive committees; the Care Group Motivators and the leaders of the Project; Dr P.H. Jaques and Dr S.P.S. Lakhana, Medical Superintendents of Elim Hospital; members of the local government and village chiefs; those who were our teachers in special courses, and many friends. They all shared their talents and knowledge with us and with the community, to the benefit of the Care Groups. Special thanks go to our families and friends who continued to encourage us to keep on, also at times when it was tough and discouraging. Two amongst them who deserve special mention are Paul Muthebule and Mavila Kwaimane, who both gave valuable advice when Selina needed it, and looked after Selina's family during the year she spent studying in Manchester.

The Care Group Project is also grateful to institutions and organisations both inside and outside South Africa for support and encouragement. Financial and material support for various projects was provided by the *Christoffel Blindenmission* (CBM) of Germany and Switzerland, and the *Département Missionnaire des Eglises Protestantes*, in Switzerland. Under the Apartheid Government, the Health Department of former Gazankulu not only allowed the Project freedom to develop its work, but paid the salaries of most of the Motivators. Now, the Health Department of the Northern Province, South Africa, is not only continuing to pay the salaries, but is actively promoting the Care Groups' aims.

This book would not have been written without the support of Professor Marcel Tanner, Director of the Swiss Tropical Institute, who insisted on the importance of publishing our experience for a wider audience which seldom has the opportunity to hear the views of the health workers at 'grass-roots' level. He supported the production of this book in many ways, and especially by suggesting the right person, Jennifer Jenkins, to edit the text. Jennifer did an excellent job by turning a rather clumsy draft into a well subdivided, easily comprehensible and readable book, and in writing and rewriting the Postscript to bring together the very different contributions of the three authors. Finally we should like to thank Christine Waslander, of KIT Publishers, Amsterdam, for her confidence in the book, and for her work in carrying it through to the final stages of production.

Many friends and colleagues have helped in the preparation of the book. We thank the many friends who read earlier versions of the manuscript and made valuable comments and suggestions, especially Barbara Müller and Vreni Schneider. Theo Schneider was most helpful in checking the words of the Tsonga proverbs and songs, and Patrick Harries revised the historical passages.

The illustrations came from many sources. We are grateful to friends who contributed photographs – which we have acknowledged wherever possible – and to Victoria Francis, who made the drawing on page 91. We have also used some of her drawings from the earlier book, *Hanyane, a Village Struggles for Eye Health*, with the permission of the co-authors. The maps were drawn by Ueli Knecht. Some of the illustrations in the Appendix are taken from the Care Group magazine, with permission from the Care Groups.

We should like to thank a number of organisations for financial support for the publication of this book, especially the Carl Schlettwein Foundation, Basel; the *Freie Akademische Gesellschaft*, Basel; the *Christoffel Blindenmission* of Switzerland and Germany; the *Schweizerischer Fonds zur Verhütung und Bekämpfung der Blindheit*, of the Swiss Ophthalmological Society; Lions International, Basel, and the *Département Missionnaire*, Switzerland. Without their help, it would not have been possible to produce this book, and distribute it at a reasonable price in countries where resources are scarce.

Selina Maphorogo and *Erika Sutter*

Preface

Why write another book on community health?

Erika Sutter

It is almost an axiom today that sustainable programmes in primary health care need community participation. Indeed, in recent years the term 'Community Based Health Care' has come into widespread use. But when books are written about projects in community health, they rarely come from the 'grass-roots' health workers, the people who have to turn ideas and goals into practice, who confront the day-to-day difficulties, and who learn a great deal about how to work with and motivate community groups. Their experience and insights are valuable, but their voices have rarely been heard.

Awareness of the processes that are taking place in the community when interventions are initiated can provide the key to their success. The workers at the grass roots know what is happening, but all too often this knowledge remains untapped. Very often, the 'establishment' does not take those lower down in the hierarchy seriously. They may even be considered as 'children', to be supervised and given orders, not as people who might have something to teach their superiors. As a result of this attitude – and of the fact that they may be vulnerable to reprisals if they question the orders received – subordinate employees seldom inform the health management about their difficulties and experiences in carrying out their tasks.

The health workers at the grass roots also find themselves caught between the 'fast-tracking' health service managers and professionals, and the slowly-progressing communities. The managers of health programmes have a task-oriented, time-oriented and outcome-oriented approach. They expect their community health workers to reach set objectives within specified time-limits. However, they tend to forget that true community participation, which should include decision-making, must be given time and cannot be rushed.

The time-frame is one problem. Another is that often project managers do not appreciate that the first step has to be the translation of the task into a process. This job is left entirely to the health workers in the community. Most of them have not been trained for it – indeed, if they are nursing assistants, low down in the hierarchical structure of the nursing system, they have often actually been discouraged from taking their own decisions. Nevertheless, as they struggle to perform the task they have been given, many grass-roots workers do learn a great deal about the process of putting ideas into practice. They are part of the community where they work, and have a profound understanding of the people's way of living and thinking that outsiders can rarely acquire.

This book is an attempt to transmit some of the insights and understanding of 'grass-roots' community health workers. The author, Selina Maphorogo, would still describe herself as one of them, but unlike many of the others, she has had the courage and the opportunity to talk about their experience and their situation. She has worked for the Elim Care Group Project for more than 25 years, and she tells the story of the growth and development of the movement as she saw and experienced it, with its successes and its frustrations.

The Project was initiated when I was head of the Eye Department of Elim Hospital, originally with the specific objective of reducing blindness. It grew rapidly into a widespread movement of groups of women working voluntarily to promote health and development in their own localities. Its most distinctive feature is the emphasis on group action rather than on individual community health workers. When the Project started, Selina Maphorogo was working as a nursing assistant in the hospital. She was asked to join the team as an interpreter, but she soon began to play a more and more important role in the Project, eventually becoming its main leader. Her understanding of both the local culture and the need for changes which would lead to better health, and her special charisma in working with people, helped to shape the way in which the Care Groups developed, and contributed very largely to their success.

At the beginning, Selina was as much a pupil as a teacher of the Care Groups and the people in the community. She was one of them, and was accepted as a respected equal. Her account thus provides a unique inside view of community action. As the project developed, and the women's awareness grew, Selina's own understanding of community dynamics deepened and her self-confidence unfolded.

Gradually, during the 8 years when I was directing the Care Group Project, the doctor/ assistant nurse relationship between Selina and myself changed to one of partnership and friendship, and she began to share her problems and experiences with me, the 'Eye Doctor'. She told me her story bit by bit as we travelled together over the rough bush roads to visit the women's health groups in remote settlements, or in the evenings in one of our homes, as we sat and discussed project and personal problems. From this, I learned more about the people to whom I had dedicated my life as a fraternal worker in a medical mission than I had learned during the previous 20 years I had lived in the area. I began to record and write down these conversations.

After I left South Africa and started teaching courses on Community Health and Development I realised that Selina's description of her experiences offered a lot of valuable information, both for teaching and for people working in similar projects.

To make the record as complete as possible, on a return visit to South Africa I recorded extensive interviews with Selina. Since it is so important for people working for the well-being of a community, whether as managers or as workers at the 'grass roots', to hear the voices and opinions of the people they wish to serve, we decided to publish this material as a book. It is our hope that those who read it will be stimulated to accept health or development workers with little formal education, but much experience, as partners – and that some of the insights and experiences described will be useful to others in their project planning.

The bulk of the book is Selina Maphorogo's story, based on our recorded interviews, and on conversations and discussions over many years. This large collection of spoken material naturally needed editing, to make a continuous narrative, to reduce the amount of repetition, and to improve clarity. However, we have tried as far as possible to ensure that the story is still told in Selina's own words. Occasional notes for readers not familiar with the project are printed in italics. We have also added a first chapter, 'Setting the Scene', and a 'Postscript'. The former describes the background to the Care Group Project, and tells the story of how it was initiated. The aim of the 'Postscript' is to set the story in a wider context and discuss the implications of Selina's story for other projects in other places. It was written together with Peter Kok, a founder member of the Care Group Project, and Carel

IJsselmuiden, who took over the Project when I left Elim in 1984. An Appendix includes a short bibliography, a glossary, and some practical information.

This book is the product of the work of many people. Many friends and colleagues gave their time to read the earlier drafts and make suggestions, and others contributed illustrations. But above all, the book is a homage to the Care Group members, and to the strength of the women of the rural areas of Africa, who are so often the main actors in making life worth living in their impoverished societies.

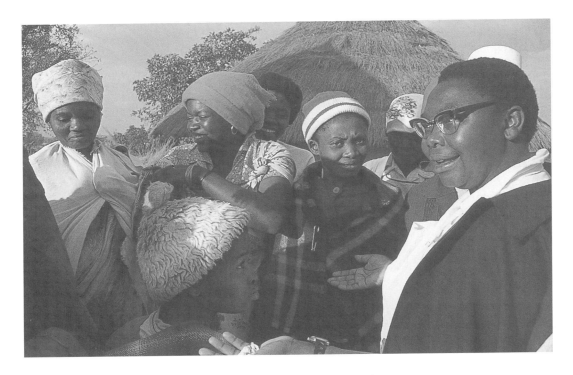

Selina and the first Care Group in 1976. (Photo: E. Sutter)

Setting the Scene

Erika Sutter

South Africa, showing
the Northern Province.
(Drawn by U. Knecht)

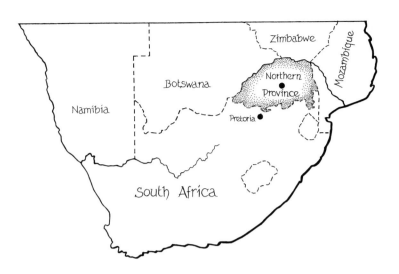

The Northern Province, showing Elim Hospital and the area of the former
'Homeland', Gazankulu. (Drawn by U. Knecht)

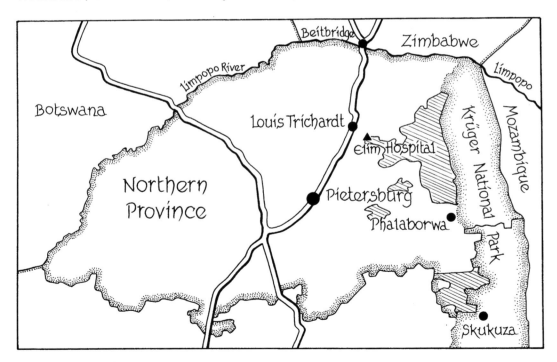

 Gazankulu

Setting the Scene

Erika Sutter

1. The country where Selina lives

When you travel from Zimbabwe to Elim you cross the Limpopo river at Beitbridge to enter South Africa, and go on driving south through the lush forest covering the southern slopes of the Soutpansberg. After an hour or two the wide plain of the Levubye valley opens before you. Descending the road to the foot of the mountain, you arrive at the little town of Louis Trichardt, with its abundance of churches and shops. It is the trading and social centre for the farmers in this north-eastern corner of South Africa.

Leaving the town, you will find a road crossing the valley that leads to Elim Hospital, 25 kilometres to the south-east. It passes through thornbush country, with cattle ranches and occasional irrigated fields growing cash crops, mainly peanuts or maize. Here and there, a farmhouse can be seen in the distance. Further to the east are vast expanses of tea, citrus, mango, pineapple or avocado plantations. But if you keep to the Elim road you cannot miss the white buildings of Elim Hospital, surrounded by tall trees, on the slope of one of the foothills of the Spelonken Range.

Before reaching the hospital on the hill, you pass by a large settlement. The round, grass-roofed houses and a few rectangular buildings with corrugated iron roofs are tightly packed along the sides of the small sandy paths. This densely populated area is an abrupt change from the land of the White farmers, with its irrigated fields and sparse population. The soil is bare and sandy; goats are busy eating the scanty dry grass that grows between the scattered low thorny bushes. You have entered 'African' country – until recently a so-called 'Homeland'.

Life is busy here in front of the hospital gate. A colourful, noisy market lines the road, where fruit, buns and even clothes are sold. Next to it is the bus and taxi station, and a bit further on a shop and a café. Further to the west is Elim church, surrounded by the houses of Elim village. Behind the hospital, in a small side valley, is a sprawling 'location', where some of the hospital staff have their homes. It is surprisingly different from the drab locations around Johannesburg, with rows of 'match-box' houses. Here, each house is different, according to the owner's imagination and financial means. There are dwellings ranging from shacks and small square houses to stately buildings. The location has a post office, a police station and some schools, but no shops. Selina Maphorogo's home, near the eastern end, can be recognised by its lush vegetable garden, and the tree nursery behind the house.

South of the hospital, a dirt road climbs up the hill. Another surprise is waiting for you when you reach the top. Far below, the wide expanse of the *lowveld* – the lowland plain – opens before you. You can hear voices coming from the many villages of round grass-roofed houses. The whole area is densely populated, teeming with children. Near the villages there are some small fields with maize – which is not thriving very well – and usually some pumpkins or beans growing between the rows. This is the area served by Elim Hospital.

In the evening, the smoke and smell of the cooking fires lies over the settlements. But life is not as cosy as it might appear. The people are fighting with inadequate resources against the odds of an arid climate, with unpredictable rainfall during the hot summer, between October and February, and dry, cool winters. The rainfall is low, averaging 400-700 mm per annum, and there are frequent prolonged periods of drought, lasting for many years – and occasional devastating floods when houses crumble and are washed away and the meagre crops are destroyed. Most rivers are dry in winter. The land, thornbush savannah, is best suited for grazing; in most areas the soil is too poor for crop farming.

The historical background

South Africa is a country of contrasts: Black / White; rich / poor; urban / rural; 'first world' / 'third world'. There is a vast gulf between the grinding poverty mainly found amongst the African population, and the immense wealth enjoyed mainly by Whites. A short excursion into the past of South Africa will explain these discrepancies.

In 1562, sailors of the Dutch East India Company landed at the Cape of Good Hope to establish a halfway station to provision their ships bound for Batavia with fresh fruit and vegetables. Dutch farmers soon settled in the area, making a living by providing the passing ships with fresh food. The original inhabitants were the semi-nomadic San and Khoikhoi, hunter-gatherers and pastoralists. After the arrival of the Dutch they were decimated by disease, and the survivors were subjected to the rule of the Company. Over the centuries, the descendants of the original Dutch settlers remained predominantly farmers. They were commonly called 'Boers' from their own word for farmer, but they themselves prefer the name, 'Afrikaners', as their home country is South Africa. Their language, Afrikaans, is an old form of Dutch, mixed with elements from French and German, and from African languages.

In 1806 the British occupied the Cape Colony (for the second time) and introduced new, more liberal laws which the Dutch disliked, so in 1827 many Boers decided to move to the north to escape British rule. On their way, they encountered Bantu-speaking Africans, living in well-organised, self-sufficient agricultural societies headed either by a chief or a king. They fought against the encroaching settlers, but were finally conquered. The British, too, expanded their territory north-eastwards. By the middle of the 19th century, most of what is known today as South Africa had been colonised by the Boers and the British.

The last independent chiefdom to be conquered was that of the Venda, living on the northern border of South Africa in the Soutpansberg mountains and their southern foothills. The Venda were not finally defeated until 1898. Only a year later, in 1899, the first Swiss missionary doctor in South Africa, Georges Liengme, started work at Elim, where a mission station had been founded for the Tsonga people three years earlier by Swiss Presbyterian missionaries. Elim Hospital was one of the first three hospitals in the whole of South Africa serving African people.

Elim lies between three tribal regions. Around the mission settlement and to the south-east, in the lowlands, are the Tsonga (also called Shangan). The Venda are mainly to the north-east, and the Pedi, or northern Sotho, to the west. In 1936 these tribal areas became part of the so-called 'Native Reserves' – the 13% of South African territory which was set aside for 80% of the total population, the

Africans. With over-population, over-grazing and subsequent soil erosion the reserves rapidly became impoverished.

The Apartheid era 1948–1994

In 1948 the Afrikaner-dominated (White only) Nationalist Government took over. They stayed in power until 1994. Their state philosophy was 'Apartheid', which means separateness of the different races; the Whites (or Europeans), the Asiatics, the Coloureds and the Africans (called 'Bantu' by the government). From that time on, a person's destiny was determined by the colour of his or her skin. The darker one was, the less chance one had of getting on in life. For the Africans, Apartheid brought with it a plethora of discriminatory laws, increasing oppression, a denial of political rights, and strict social and geographical separation along colour lines.

In pursuit of the policy of separation, the members of ten indigenous African tribes were segregated into 'pure' ethnic groups. Each group was assigned its own territory, and people who lived in the 'wrong' area were forcibly relocated. The territories were within the restricted area of the old Native Reserves, which were only minimally enlarged. The relocation process robbed 2–3 million people of their land, their livelihood and their jobs, causing untold suffering. These territories were first called 'Homelands', then 'National States'. They were popularly (and ironically) known as 'Bantustans'. A puppet government was installed in each 'Homeland' under the strict supervision of the White government in Pretoria, and the residents were given some political rights – but only within the 'Homeland' itself.

With a few exceptions the 'Homelands' consisted of several portions of land, with areas assigned to other ethnic groups in between, forming a crazy pattern. In the northern region, the 'Homelands' Lebowa (for the Pedi), Venda (for the Venda), and Gazankulu (for the Tsonga) were so intertwined that a journey of a few kilometres might easily cross territories of all three 'Bantustans' as well as White-owned land. This distribution of land led to numerous disputes between the previously well-integrated ethnic groups, and disrupted community life in the whole region.

The Nationalist Government revived tribalism in order to 'divide and rule'. When the autonomous chiefdoms were conquered by the advancing European settlers in the 19th century, the local chiefs in most areas lost much of their power. The Nationalist Government tried to restore their status to some extent, so that at the local level many settlements were administered by chiefs or headmen and their councillors. *De facto*, however, the chiefdoms had not really become autonomous again, but were ruled by the White government in Pretoria through its Native Commissioners. The powers of the tribal authorities were reduced to land allocation, the settling of minor disputes, tax collection and the day-to-day running of their area. Chiefs who opposed the Apartheid line were removed. Yet the chiefs still had a considerable grip on their subjects – which could have both good and bad results – and the villagers had to adjust to this. They could not be ignored when community programmes were introduced (as is made clear in the later chapters of the book).

The Apartheid regime did to a large extent achieve its aim of separating people of different races. Selina was five years old when the Nationalist Government came to power, so throughout her childhood and most of her adult life this was the society she knew. For her, it was the normal state of affairs. It was unusual to have contacts like those she and her family had with the Swiss staff at the hospital, who (like many foreign missionaries) often ignored the Apartheid laws. Normally, Africans used to keep at a safe distance from Whites, who generally were not to be trusted.

This historical outline is important in setting the scene for the story of the Care Groups. It is, of course, vastly over-simplified. The picture that emerges tends to be one of the 'good' African and the 'bad' White – but of course not all Africans are 'poor and good', and there have always been many Whites, both of Boer and British ancestry, who have sincerely cared for the Africans – though often in a rather paternalistic mode. This also becomes clear from Selina's story, which includes actors of many nationalities and colours.

Gazankulu

Gazankulu no longer exists, but as most of the story told in this book happened between 1976 and 1996, this is the name that we have generally used to refer to the region. Gazankulu was the name given to the Tsonga 'Homeland', in which Elim hospital and Selina's home were situated. With the abolition of Apartheid in 1994, when the 'Homelands' were dismantled and reintegrated into South Africa, the area became part of the Northern Province.

In the 'Homeland' the Apartheid government enforced its 'betterment' scheme. The traditional scattered settlements, where extended families lived in clusters of houses surrounded by their fields, were replaced by large closed township-type residential areas, without property rights. With the prevailing lack of sanitation, this form of settlement became a health hazard. Furthermore, this change made 60% of the population landless, and the remainder obtained inadequate plots, so that subsistence farming was replaced by a poor consumer economy. People complained that 'Disease and crime travel fast along the new straight roads.' There was often only one water outlet for 700–1000 people, usually at a distance from the settlement. Women carried the water, which was mainly used for drinking and cooking, in 25-litre containers on their heads. Only in recent years was water installed in a large number of settlements, with one standpipe per 10–20 households.

Gazankulu, with a population of 700 000 or more, was one of the poorest homelands. Job opportunities existed for only 10% of the inhabitants of working age. Consequently, about 60% of the able-bodied men were working as migrant labourers in the big cities, and were absent from home most of the year, often only returning at Christmas for the yearly renewal of their labour contracts. Their families were prohibited from following the breadwinner to town. The permanent population therefore consisted predominantly of women and children. The men who remained – apart from a few with jobs in local government or the health services, and a few with small businesses like shopkeepers and taxi-owners – were the elderly, the sick, and the unemployed. The prevalent diseases in the region were those typical of a deprived society: malnutrition, bilharzia, gastro-enteritis, typhoid fever, measles, tuberculosis and the blinding eye disease trachoma. Later, HIV/AIDS became the biggest health hazard.

Schooling was neither compulsory nor free, and of those children who did attend school, a great number dropped out after one or two years, either because there was no money for school fees, or because boys had to look after the cattle and girls had to help at home. For a long time, people did not think it important that girls should be educated. Literacy was therefore especially low amongst women, being around 40%, though it gradually improved to 60%. Most of the schools, especially secondary schools, were originally run by foreign missions. In these schools English had been introduced early on and had reached a good standard. However, in 1952, at the time Selina was attending primary school, the mission schools had been nationalised and the Bantu Education Act enforced. This meant inferior schooling. Africans were supposed to remain cheap unskilled labourers satisfying the White economy. At best, they could become nurses, teachers or officials for their own ethnic group. Teaching was in the vernacular for the first 8 years, and afterwards half in Afrikaans and half in English, with a few subjects still in the vernacular. The result was a rapid decline in proficiency in the English language.

2. Elim Hospital and its Health Ward

Elim Hospital, founded in 1899 by the Swiss Presbyterian mission, is the biggest and oldest hospital in the region, with 600 beds. About 15 years later a Scottish mission hospital was built in the mountains of Vendaland, 70 kilometres to the east. Until the period 1940–1950, when three more hospitals were established, these two hospitals were the only ones catering for a population of over 2 million.

Elim hospital consists of a complex of bungalow-style buildings, housing medical, surgical, paediatric and maternity sections, a ward for tuberculosis patients and one for chronic patients. In 1933, an ophthalmic section was added. Up to 1948 this was the only place in the Transvaal Province where eye care was available for Africans, and it still caters for a population of approximately 2 million. A school for a post-basic course for the Diploma in Ophthalmic Nursing was opened in 1975. At the time when Selina worked there, the Eye Section had about 100 beds. Due to the nature of ophthalmology as a speciality of its own, requiring specially trained staff, the Eye Section has always been a separate little kingdom, where contact with the generalists, doctors as well as nurses, remained limited.

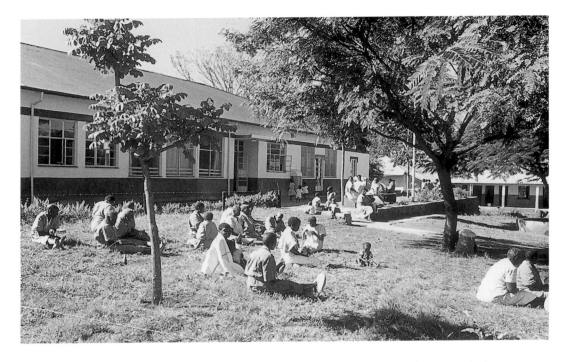

Eye patients enjoying the sun in front of the Eye Department, Elim Hospital.
(Photo: E. Sutter)

As Elim is situated between three tribal areas, patients from all
three ethnic groups, the Tsonga, the Venda and the Pedi, have always
regarded it as *their* hospital. It was therefore a shock when, in 1979,
the Government decreed that each 'Homeland' would have its own
Health Department, and every hospital and clinic was supposed to
cater exclusively for its 'own' ethnic group. This meant, for example,
that Venda patients who lived in the western part of their
'Homeland' were supposed to go to a Venda hospital 30 kilometres
east of Elim. On the way – unless they ignored the new rules, as
many patients did – they went right past Elim Hospital, which they
had always attended in the past. With the new Health Departments,
the health system had to be reorganised, and each hospital was
allocated an area in which it was responsible for both curative and
preventive care. These areas were called Health Wards.

Steps from the hospital into the community

Elim Hospital has a longer tradition of community involvement than any of the other hospitals in the northern region. By the 1950s, clinics ('Health Points') had already been established over a wide area, reaching as far as almost 100 kilometres to the east as well as to the west, but after the administrative changes described above, all the clinics outside the Elim Hospital Health Ward were taken over by other hospitals.

In the early 1970s, some of the more progressive doctors in Elim became concerned about health in the community outside the hospital, and carried out surveys of child health and other topics. The Eye Section staff joined them to do population surveys on trachoma. The people in the villages got used to doctors and medical students visiting them, and on the whole they appreciated their efforts. However, these early interventions met with many obstacles from other quarters. Many colleagues, and the hospital management, failed to understand why doctors should want to spend time on this kind of work. Furthermore, at that time the South African Government viewed all community involvement with suspicion, seeing it as potentially tainted with communism.

One of the doctors, who became very much involved in this work, Peter Kok from the Netherlands, has contributed his personal story (Box 1). He describes his reactions as a doctor arriving fresh from Europe and being faced with a situation of ill-health that he had never met before, and his surprise at the local people who had come to see these diseases of poverty as 'normal'. He also writes about his anger and distress at the initially unsympathetic response of the hospital management and most of his colleagues to his efforts to introduce preventive care in the communities. However, it was not long before the same hospital management team became staunch and reliable supporters of community involvement by hospital staff. It was much harder to convince colleagues trained in high-quality curative medicine of the value of preventive and promotive care. These colleagues felt that they had been left with all the real work, while those doing community surveys were just enjoying themselves, ambling around in their cars and chatting with a few people here and there.

Box 1: Moving into the community

Contributed by Dr Peter Kok, who went to work in Elim Hospital in the 1970s.

Being confronted with children in various states of malnutrition, from the marasmic child to the one with a swollen body, cold sores and a destroyed cornea, made a deep impression on us young doctors. We soon felt that optimal treatment at an academic level left much unsaid between us. Where were all these children coming from? Were the children we saw just a fraction of the whole, like the nose of a hippo surfacing above the dark waters ... ?

For the nurses, perhaps, these children were a normal part of the patient population – and malnutrition was even something that was so common in the communities they came from that it did not arouse the same curiosity as it did in us new doctors. We became more and more anxious to see for ourselves what was going on outside the hospital. We were already visiting some of the outlying health clinics regularly, but we only saw the sick and hardly met the community.

We presented our worries about the severity of the malnutrition problem in the children's ward (60% were malnourished!) to the management of the hospital, and requested assistance to do a community survey. Our request was met by an incomprehensible 'No'. We doctors were told we had been recruited for medical work in the hospital and were not supposed to go into the villages to do investigations. What for? In the politically sensitive situation of the time, any attempt by foreigners to go into the communities was met by official suspicion. The management thought it highly risky to reveal facts about the nutritional status of children in South Africa, lest the world might know! How could children in a country with such an abundance of food for export, able to feed half of the African continent, not feed its own children?

The only way around this 'No' was to organise the survey in our time off. One Saturday afternoon we left in our private cars with one friendly and daring nurse to go to a small place 50 km from the hospital and do our survey. We found people most interested in being examined at the local clinic free of charge, and hundreds of children were examined, weighed and measured. Nearly all of the 300 children in the village were brought to the clinic. We learned several new things. Firstly, that people were willing to come for a survey when it was properly prepared by the local nurse and organised through the village leadership. Secondly, that 22% of the children were underweight, and 3% seriously malnourished – 1 % with kwashiorkor.

But we still did not understand at all why the children were in that state. One question answered led to 10 unanswered questions.

We also learned that people did not listen to the taped health messages coming from our loudspeaker and our small battery-operated tape recorder. We found that most mothers also wanted to be examined, and many presented with often serious pellagra. In short, the survey left us with data, but no solutions to the community problems we found.

We had most likely raised expectations in the community that we were going to help them with these problems. Doing nothing after such a manifestation of community awareness of health issues is not acceptable, even if it does often happen! In our case, a fortnightly visit to the same clinic, building up a good relationship with the nurse, eventually created a solid bond between hospital and community, and opened the way for an exchange of knowledge.

Teaching the mothers to feed their children in a better, 'scientific' way with high-calorie locally available food was undertaken at every opportunity when a captive audience waiting for the clinic doors to open presented itself. The teaching was of the good straightforward type which people were used to in the church: somebody preaching above them and talking over their heads. It was much later that we learned to really talk *with* people.

It was on one such occasion that a mother stood up and said, 'How can we give our children more meat when our chickens are falling dead from the trees?' The group of women around her supported her view, and more were coming forward to air the same. What can a doctor trained in human health do for chickens? To gain credibility, I went off to the nearest town and consulted a veterinary surgeon who informed me that the deaths were probably caused by Newcastle disease, and all the chickens should be vaccinated. The similarity with us immunising thousands of children to protect their health became suddenly apparent. Why could doctors not protect people's health by immunising their chickens?

Again there was resistance at the hospital, when we mentioned an activity so far away from academic medicine. Who has ever heard of doctors grabbing chicken after chicken and immunising them for the sake of healthy children? Nevertheless, we did it – and the people were happy. We had done something to solve what they had perceived as their problem. And, after that, teaching a local person to continue immunising chickens was easy.

Increasing emphasis on community health

In the 1970s, the Government introduced a comprehensive health system, which included curative, preventive, promotive and rehabilitative care, and laid somewhat more emphasis on community health. Each hospital was made responsible for the outreach services in its Health Ward, providing staff and materials for the clinics and ensuring that doctors visited them regularly. The clinics catered for minor ailments, mother and child health, and preventive care. The system brought an improvement in the integration of curative and preventive care, though some hospitals continued to neglect services at the periphery.

Over the years, the health services at the periphery were extended and some clinics were replaced by Health Centres with better equipment and staff. However, many people still had to travel long distances to reach a clinic – for example, the Elim Health Ward had clinics only in approximately every fifth or sixth settlement. In the 1980s, Community Health Workers (CHWs), chosen by their communities and trained to the level of nursing assistants, were introduced to serve the villages where there was no clinic. In addition, these settlements received monthly visits from a mobile clinic to provide a predominantly preventive service. The community members were encouraged to participate in running health services through clinic advisory committees, whose members were local people; usually some teachers, some councillors and the chief. Men were generally in the majority.

Public Health Nurses based in the hospitals were responsible for the clinics and the CHWs, and were the contact persons between the committees and the hospital. Other aspects of public health were the responsibility of the Area Health Inspectors. They inspected food shops and water supplies, and were in charge of the sanitary workers who checked the erection of toilets and the water sources, and sprayed the houses against mosquitoes before the malaria season. They also supervised the work of the Health Educators who carried out vaccination campaigns, tuberculosis control and health education, for example in schools.

It was during the period of change and reorganisation in the 1970s, at a time when the institutional health services had little contact with many villages, that the Care Group Movement started. The Care Groups – groups of women, working as unpaid volunteers –

quickly became important actors in the effort to foster community health. The initiative to start a community project came from individuals working in Elim Hospital, but once the work had gained momentum the hospital management started to release some staff to help to organise the groups and train the members. As the Care Group Movement expanded and the activities became more diverse it developed an organisation of its own, and a lot of financial support came from outside donors. However, the link to the public Health Services remained, and most of the Motivators are still Health Service employees.

As public health interventions expanded, it became increasingly difficult to co-ordinate the different activities and people working for health in the community. The Public Health Nurses, the Health Educators and the Care Group Motivators all had their offices in different buildings, in three corners of the hospital grounds, so that they hardly met except at the hospital's monthly staff meetings. Each section did its own work without much communication with the others, which led to duplication, and confused the public. The situation improved when all the offices were united in one building, the Community Health Office, and weekly planning meetings were arranged.

3. The Care Groups

The early days – trachoma control

The Care Group movement grew from a project that was originally initiated with the limited objective of controlling the eye disease trachoma (Box 2). Trachoma was one of the most common causes of blindness in the area around Elim Hospital in the 1970s, and our surveys showed that on average almost 50% of children aged 2–4 years were severely affected by the disease in its most infective stage. Most of them lived in the most poverty stricken sections of the villages where personal and environmental hygiene was weak. In contrast, in the better-off families, like those of teachers, shopkeepers or taxi owners, we found only a few mild cases of trachoma.

Box 2: Trachoma

Trachoma is a communicable, preventable eye disease, linked to poverty and to inadequate personal and environmental hygiene. The disease occurs predominantly in arid areas in the southern hemisphere. It is transmitted from eye to eye by direct contact or by flies, within the family and the neighbourhood. In areas of high endemicity, even the very young children are already affected. In this age group the causative agent (the bacterium *Chlamydia trachomatis*) is at its most virulent, reaching its peak between the ages of 2–4 years. When unsatisfactory hygienic conditions favour the spread of the disease, the young children are the main transmitters within their immediate surroundings, and represent the main reservoir of infection in a community. They pass the infection on to their siblings, mothers and grandmothers. Spontaneous cure tends to occur by the time the children reach school age. A single infection, followed by cure, does not cause any harm to the eyes. But many years of repeated rein-fections later in life eventually lead to the blinding complications, corneal scarring and entropion (in-turning of the eyelashes) leading to further scarring.

It follows that the best strategy to control blinding trachoma in a community is to create an environment that prevents reinfection by improving hygiene and reducing the number of flies. This can be supported by antibiotic treatment of pre-school children and others with severe infections, which will decrease the infective load in a locality. However, our surveys have proved that simply improving hygienic conditions, even without antibiotic treatment, can significantly reduce the prevalence of trachoma.

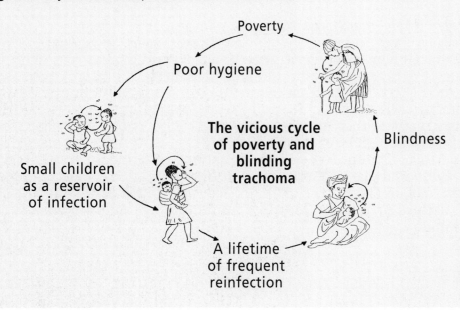

Poverty

Poor hygiene

The vicious cycle
of poverty and
blinding
trachoma

Blindness

Small children
as a reservoir
of infection

A lifetime
of frequent
reinfection

It is repeated reinfection over many years that leads eventually to blindness. Infection spreads from the young children through direct eye-to-eye transmission by touch, soiled cloths, or flies. It was thus not surprising that it was amongst those tending young children in the poor families – the older siblings, the mothers and the grandmothers – that we found most of the blinding complications of trachoma. Men were much less affected than women. As migrant labourers they were absent from their homes most of the time, and even if they were at home they traditionally left the care of their children to the women.

At that time, the most frequently used measure to control trachoma was mass treatment of schoolchildren with tetracycline eye ointment, but this would clearly not help in communities where the main transmitters were the pre-school children. We concluded that we had to attend to the root causes of trachoma, which lay in the people's everyday environment. We needed to prevent reinfection by motivating the people to improve hygienic conditions in their homes and surroundings, and to reduce the infective load in the community by treating the young children. At that time, only a fraction of small children were brought to child health clinics. So not only the improvement of hygiene, but also the treatment of the children, would have to be done by the mothers. We had to aim at active participation of the people in the affected communities, especially women.

Trachoma infection spreads from young children, e.g. through flies, and leads to repeated reinfection and blindness in the family. (Photo: E. Sutter)

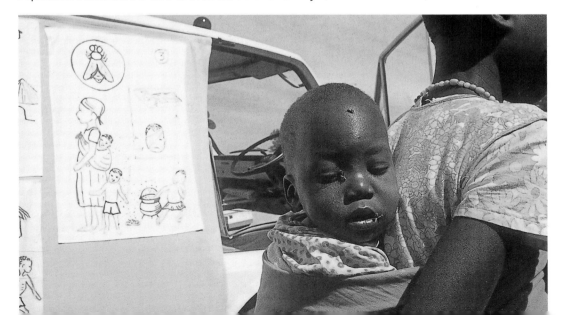

Repeated infection leads to
blindness later in life. In-turning
of the eyelashes (entropion)
causes corneal scarring.
(Photo: L. Lawson)

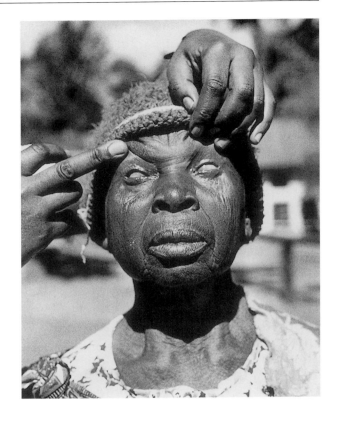

A first trial of this concept was started in 1975 by staff members
from Elim Hospital. The 'Trachoma Team' consisted of myself
(Erika Sutter) as the ophthalmologist; Dr Peter Kok from Holland;
a community health worker; the hospital's medical superintendent,
and three ophthalmic nursing students. An especially needy
settlement was chosen, which was one of the worst places for
trachoma. It was some 30 km from the hospital, and could only be
reached along poor roads. The key persons – chiefs and teachers –
were approached for permission to work in their village, and the
local women's club agreed to help. Health workers from the
hospital screened all the households for trachoma and gave health
education. The members of the women's club were instructed
about the nature of the disease, how it spread, and how it could be
prevented. They were shown how to apply the tetracycline eye
ointment, and were provided with a supply of it. They were to
treat all the positive cases identified by the health workers, and
their contacts, and to reinforce the health education. The scheme
appeared to be well accepted by the community.

However, soon after the initial phase the summer rains started, and the roads became impassable, preventing any monitoring of the programme. By the time we could visit the place again, the ointment had been used up – but the people in the poor section of the village, where trachoma was severe, had not received any treatment. The members of the women's club had refused to go to the 'dirty' people living there. The villagers were no longer interested in the scheme, despite the goodwill of the teachers, who had included trachoma education in the school programme.

We had started with only very rudimentary knowledge about community involvement in health care, and we had to ask ourselves what had gone wrong. We realised that firstly, the project was imposed from outside. The team from the hospital had obtained permission from the village authorities, but the people concerned had no say. Secondly, we had not been aware of the social division in the community. Using the 'educated, clean' people to attend to the 'uneducated, dirty' people had aggravated the schism. The members of the women's club belonged to the higher social class in the community, where trachoma was not a problem, and therefore they had no vested interest in the project. Finally, we realised that in very poor communities, where most people have to struggle simply to make ends meet, there is not much time or energy to respond to a new venture.

Having learned these lessons, we made a new attempt in 1976. This time, three settlements were chosen where people were already active in community development – for example, where there were church women's groups, or literacy projects. We hoped that people in these communities would respond positively, and that we would gain experience that would make it easier to continue elsewhere. The new team consisted of myself, the ophthalmic nurses, and Selina Maphorogo, who was working as a nursing assistant in the Eye Department, as interpreter.

We started by asking the village authorities in each community to organise a mass meeting, where the problem of trachoma was discussed. Naturally the first reaction was to suggest that health professionals – preferably the doctor – should attend to the problem. When, after lengthy discussions, the people understood that they themselves could do the job much better, 15–20 women in each settlement and an occasional man offered to help. From the beginning, the idea was that the Care Groups would function like other women's organisations in the area, with the members working voluntarily. We therefore made it clear that there would be no remuneration for work done. The reward would be a healthy family and community.

It became evident in the first months that trained nurses were often too far away from the local culture to be able to communicate well with the village people. Assistant nurses were closer to the community, so once the first group of ophthalmic nurses had finished their training, the project relied on assistant nurses rather than on trained nurses. Selina's own story describes how she moved from passing on the health messages she had been taught to finding a better method of communication, based on a close contact with the community.

In due course, the volunteers organised themselves into groups, electing their own leaders. A name had to be found for them, and 'Care Groups' was suggested. At first, it was regarded as temporary, until the groups could come up with their own *Tsonga* name, but the name stuck, and they are called 'Care Groups' to this day. The Care Groups continued to receive training and assistance from the hospital-based team. After the first year, assistant nurses who worked in the community were released from hospital duties for Care Group work, and were called Care Group Motivators.

Selina Maphorogo was the first Care Group Motivator. She was joined by a male social worker, but the project grew so fast that the two of them could hardly cope. One village after another wanted to join with its own group. It was impossible to slow down this process, and more Motivators had to be appointed. The story Selina tells is mainly about the groups in the Elim Health Ward, but the groups also spread into other areas in Gazankulu and Venda, based on other hospitals, each of which ran the project more-or-less in its own way with its own staff.

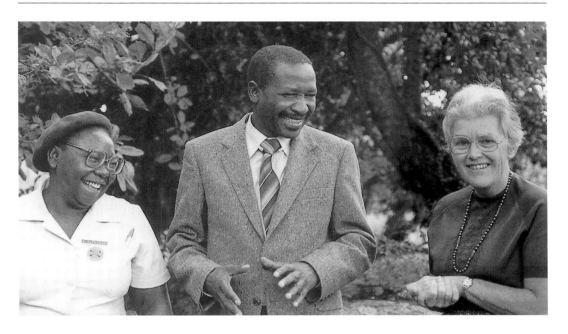

Erika Sutter with the first two Care Group Motivators, Selina Maphorogo and the social worker Andrew Radebe. (Photo: R. Collins)

Expansion and diversification

Within three years of the founding of the Care Groups, the prevalence of active trachoma had decreased by 50%, and a few years later the disease had almost disappeared from the area. Even before this point was reached, the groups had begun to concern themselves with other aspects of health, like child nutrition and vegetable growing. As time went on, other issues of village development were included in their programme. Some addressed community problems such as water supplies, or care for the aged or the disabled, or they organised crèches for children of working mothers. Others started income-generating co-operatives.

Additional funding and staff training

As the Care Group Project started as an extension service of the hospital's ophthalmic department, it was originally a governmental institution. Most of the staff were on the Government's pay roll, and for a while the hospital was able to provide some eye ointment. However, as the project grew it needed more staff and equipment than the health services could provide. It was also important to be able to respond to the groups' immediate needs, such as the provision of revolving loans for certain projects. For all this, funding was essential. Fortunately, long-term donors were found, especially the *Christoffel Blindenmission* in Germany, and the *Département Missionaire* in Switzerland. However, most of the staff are still paid by the Government, and the project remains closely linked to the regional health services. The Care Group Project is thus simultaneously part of the Government Health Services, and an NGO (non-governmental organisation). This mixed status has advantages and disadvantages. These are discussed in more detail in the last chapter of this book.

Besides the need for funds, another problem as the project grew was that of staff training. At the beginning, all the people in the team were both learners and teachers. None of them had any experience of this type of project. The doctors in charge were not even aware of the Motivators' need for systematic training, and they were given nothing but some rather haphazard brief instructions before they left for work in the mornings. Being sent into the community completely unprepared for the new venture left the first Motivators with a permanent feeling of insecurity, which could never be completely remedied by training later on.

Later, training became more systematic. Weekly in-service training sessions were introduced for the team, complemented by yearly or half-yearly refresher courses run by trainers from various development organisations. Opportunities were found for Motivators to visit courses outside the district. However, few of them took advantage of these. Selina Maphorogo was exceptional in that she was both willing to seize the opportunities offered, and able to do so because her husband and family were supportive. She even agreed to go to England for a year, to attend a course in Adult Education, Community Development and Community Health at the University of Manchester. This gave her a wider view, and enabled her to continue to lead the Care Groups into the next millennium.

4. Care Groups and community health in the New South Africa

When the new government came to power in 1994 and the 'homelands' were abolished, the health system changed radically. The colour bar disappeared. A central Ministry of Health, deciding on national policy, has replaced the 14 'ethnic' health departments of the Apartheid era. Nine provincial offices are responsible for the implementation of the national policy in the provinces, and for delegating powers to the smaller regional offices. The new regional boundaries within the provinces do not correspond at all with the previous homeland boundaries, which makes the transition extremely complicated on the local level.

There has also been a basic change in health policy. The emphasis has shifted from a predominantly curative approach to promoting Primary Health Care, and from a strongly centralised organisation to decentralisation. In the days of Apartheid, the allocation of funds heavily favoured the 20% of Whites in the population. Now the principle is equity in funds and services for all.

With the new emphasis on preventive and promotive care, more activities are being directed towards the community. There is also more emphasis on fostering a democratic spirit within the work force, with everybody having a chance to contribute to decision-making. For this purpose, innumerable meetings are called where the new approaches are supposed to be discussed.

In this new setting the Care Group Motivators should be able to make a valuable contribution, if they can succeed in making their voices heard, because in their work they have gained a lot of practical experience of democratic processes and the sharing of knowledge. In practice, it does not yet work, because the people in charge at the regional and hospital levels have grown up in an authoritative system with a strict nursing hierarchy. They are not yet used to a partnership approach, and are not ready to listen to what those 'lower down' have to say.

The Care Group Movement itself continues to flourish. It has formed its own association with a leadership of strong women from the ranks of the groups, determined to continue to pursue the aim of working towards a better quality of life for the whole of their community.

In all the health wards together, there are now approximately 250 groups comprising about 10 000 women (and a few men), and 30 Motivators. The groups have become a platform in their community where common problems are discussed and solutions sought. The women have found their identity, and they are trusted and respected as wise counsellors by their communities.

Chapter 1

Selina's story: from domestic worker to community health promoter

Matimba ya mhisi ku hlota
The strength of the hyena is in hunting
One finds what one wants by untiring efforts

Chapter 1

Selina's story: from domestic worker to community health promoter

1. Where I came from

My childhood

I was born in 1943 in Elim, in the Northern Province of South Africa. This is a Tsonga area, but my family belonged to the Venda people. My parents and my two older sisters were living in Elim because my father was employed at the hospital as a driver. After I was born I was given the Venda name *Ntame*, which means 'admire me'. The Tsonga did not understand the meaning of this name and called me Selina, and I have been known by this name ever since. My mother died of TB when I was 9 months old, and my father took care of us children. The Swiss housekeeper at the hospital used to send enough milk and baby food to our house, so that I could be fed properly. The best person in my life was my father. He was such a good person! I used to eat with him from his dish, and I tasted all the food he was eating, even meat. This is unusual in our culture, because traditionally only old people and men eat eggs and chicken. Children should not be spoiled and cry for meat. This was a very selfish culture, benefiting the men. The men used to add a lot of pepper, so that nobody else could eat the meat.

It was not easy to grow up with no mother. I did not have any grandparents who could look after me either, as my grandmother had died, leaving my grandfather alone. I had only my father. I had to adjust myself to meet whatever might come, and accept help when it was offered. Our aunt came from time to time to look after our clothes and such things. But most of the time we stayed with a good neighbour who was a very wise woman. She offered us hot food when we needed it and comforted us. She even gave better care to us than to her own children.

From early childhood I had to learn the hard way and to persevere until I succeeded. For example when I was 12 years old I decided to make a dress for myself. I did not know how to do it, but I went on struggling. I did not want to ask for help. Then someone saw what I was doing and finished the dress with me. The habit of finding my own way, and keeping on learning by myself, has remained with me throughout my life.

My father married again when I was seven years old and had started school. I was very cross at first. I could not understand what this woman was doing in our home. It was only after I understood better why he did it that I started to get on with my stepmother. From then on, I liked her very much. She taught me many things, such as picking wild vegetables, weeding, planting, and fetching wood. She had another 7 children, and I enjoyed playing with them after school. We used to act sketches and play games I learned from the 'Sunbeams', and I taught them many songs. I liked to attend the meetings of the 'Sunbeams' and later the 'Wayfarers', where we learned many useful skills and had fun with games and songs. We were also told how to behave at home, at school, with neighbours and with the elderly. On Sundays we put on our beautiful dresses to go to Sunday school. We heard about Jesus and many other Bible stories, and learned what is good and what is bad.

Most of the time as children we were playing around the hospital. At weekends, when my father was driving the Swiss nurses somewhere for a picnic, we were invited to join them. I still remember the wonderful sandwiches the nurses used to share with us. In this way I was introduced very early to the culture of the Swiss people. We knew how the whites behaved. As children, we had no idea what apartheid was.

Most of what I know about my own rural culture I learned from elderly people, for example from my grandfather. He was a traditional healer. He used to 'throw bones' in order to find out what type of medicine he must give to the patient. The people liked him, because he was a responsible and good healer. But he could not tell you who is troubling you at home and such things. He was not good at that. From my grandfather I learned a lot about herbs.

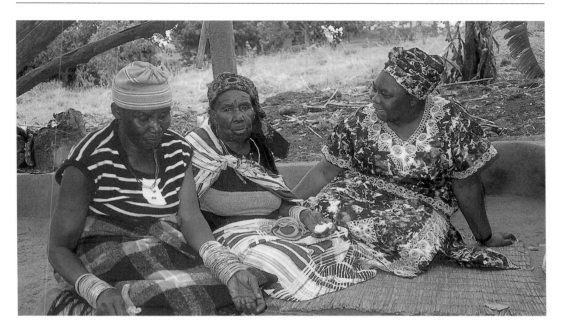

'I learned a lot about my own culture from elderly relatives, like my husband's grandmother and her family.' (Photo: E. Sutter)

What I learned then is still useful to me today. I know how to behave when I enter the house of a Venda family, how to greet and what to do, because most of my relatives belong to the Venda people. There are some valuable lessons in traditional culture. We learned that we must not eat *vuswa* (maize meal porridge) without washing our hands. We also learned that when older people were talking, children were not supposed to listen. That is the reason that also today I can have two friends who do not like each other. When I am with the one I don't talk about the other one.

My first job

I attended school for eight years, up to Standard 6, and managed to pass the examination, though learning was not easy for me. I was able to start at Lemana, the Mission secondary school, but then my father got severely ill and I had to look after him. I did washing and ironing for other people, and sold fruit. After four years my father died, leaving all 10 children behind. My two older sisters were married by then. Now I had to become independent, stop my schooling and earn a living. I became a nanny in one of the doctor's families at the hospital. I learned many new things; other methods of cooking, and a good way of caring for children. This was the first time in my life that I stayed in a white South African family. Many things were quite different from what I was used to, and they were eating things I had never seen or heard of before. So sometimes it happened that I did not understand what 'Madam' (this is what we Africans had to call the white lady of the house) wanted me to do.

A cross-cultural misunderstanding

The second Christmas I was working for that family, Madam told me: 'Selina, I bought a big chicken for you and the gardener. You can share it together for Christmas.' The gardener wanted to go home after finishing work, and I told him about the chicken. As he didn't want to wait until I cooked it, we decided to divide it. I went to the fridge and there was a very, very big chicken, as well as a medium one and a small one. I was very happy to see such a big chicken. I had never seen such a big one before. As Madam said she had bought us a big chicken, we took that one and divided it between us. At 3 o'clock Madam said, 'Selina, we have many people for supper. It is time to start roasting the turkey.' I said, 'Yes, madam' and waited for her to give me the turkey. She opened the fridge and cried, 'Where is the turkey? Where is the turkey?' I said, 'I don't know. I have only taken the big chicken you bought for us.' She was so cross with me. Since then I know what a turkey is – I had never heard of it before. Later we often laughed about that story, after we had become good friends.

My employer was also very good at gardening, and I learned a lot which is still useful for me today. This lady also discovered that there was something wrong with my eyes. I could not see well far away, and the doctor at the eye hospital ordered glasses for me. It was only then that I discovered why I could never finish taking notes at school or writing my tests. I thought I was dull. Now this was a new world for me and I was very thankful. I think if this had been discovered earlier I could have done very well at school.

Marriage, and more working experience

After the doctor and his family left the hospital in 1965 I had to stop working for a while, because I was getting married, and I had many things to organise. My husband is a builder. At that time he was looking after his mother and his three sisters. I had to find a place to make a home, which was not easy. Then I had my first child, a girl. The second girl followed soon afterwards. By that time I was working again. I had been offered a job as a privately paid primary school teacher to step in for a qualified teacher who was ill. I had to walk 10 kilometres every day because there was no transport to that school. I enjoyed teaching school children. After school I volunteered to help a missionary lady who was teaching adults who could not read and write. I taught the ladies how to sew and make clothes for their children. We also made necklaces from seeds we collected from the trees. This was a wonderful time for me. We could do all this and at the same time we were sharing our problems and skills.

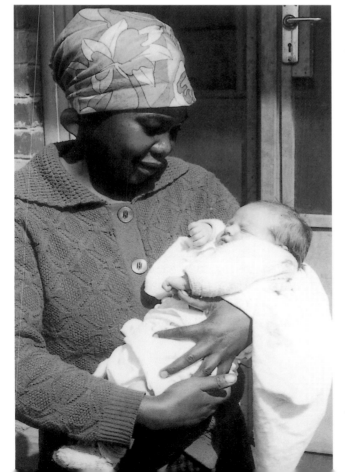

'In 1970, most of the day I looked after the Dutch doctor's baby.'
(Photo: J. Geretsen)

When the qualified teacher came back after some years, I had to stop teaching, and again got a job as domestic worker. This time it was for a Dutch couple. They were both doctors at the hospital. When they had a baby, I was the one looking after it most of the day. I liked this child very much and she got used to me. When they went on holiday, they used to take me with them to look after the baby. In this way I visited many places in South Africa I had never seen before. But there were problems with travelling because of the apartheid laws. When it came to staying a night in a hotel, I was not allowed to sleep in a room in the hotel. Even if the doctors offered for me to stay with them in their room, it was not allowed because of my black skin. I was made to sleep in an outside room with the servants, who were often very rough people, and the place was dirty and it was not safe. So sometimes I took my things and went to sleep in the car. But this was not safe either; I was so scared and could not sleep.

A job in Elim hospital

When the Dutch doctors left for Europe, I found a job in the hospital, as an interpreter for the doctors in the eye department. During that time my third girl was born. In 1973 I was allowed to attend the six-month training course for assistant nurses, where I learned about various health issues and how to look after patients. Within the structure of the nursing profession, I have remained at the grade of assistant nurse ever since, because according to the nursing regulations I would need to have passed 'matric.' to train as a nurse.

After training, I went on working in the eye department as an assistant nurse. The job was very interesting. I had to learn a lot about eye diseases. The Eye Doctor explained things to us properly, especially diseases like trachoma, cataract and glaucoma. She did not show us what an eye looks like using a slit lamp – only nursing students were allowed to look; we nursing assistants only held the patient's head. But she did show us what trachoma and pterygium look like. I was interested, and I felt that I understood about these diseases and how one could prevent some of them.

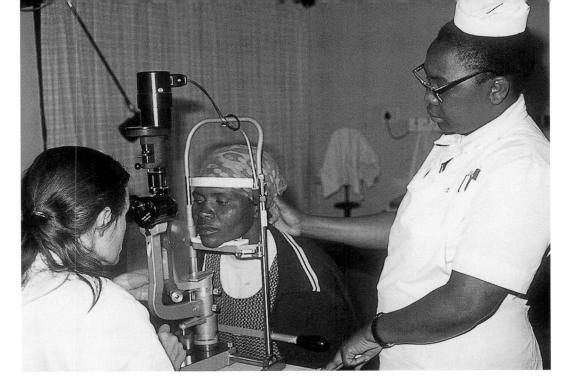

'We assistant nurses were not shown what an eye looks like at the slit lamp.
We were only holding the patient's head.' (Photo: E. Sutter)

The doctor made us explain to the patients, as well as translating
what they said to her. I managed to explain to patients with cataract
what is going to happen at the operation, and I gave health
education in the ward while the doctor was busy in the operating
theatre. We in the eye department knew that people only got the
right treatment if they told the truth, for example when we
examined their vision. We explained to the patients why they
should not guess, and that they would not be punished for not
seeing the signs on the chart properly. This was different from the
general wards, where the doctors often didn't get the true story.
The nurses did not know enough, because the doctors had no time
to explain to the nurses.

I liked to talk to the patients. One who became my special friend
was a *mufundisi* (pastor) from Mozambique. His name was Gabriel.
I was pregnant at that time, and he told me, 'It will be a boy' – and
it was a boy. This is why I called the baby Gabriel.

2. A new job; working in the community

The beginning of the Care Groups

In 1976, after I was back from maternity leave, the Eye Doctor
allocated me to a new project which had just been started. The aim
was to attack the problem of the eye disease trachoma with the
help of the community. The doctors and ophthalmic nurses who
organised the project were known as the 'Trachoma Team'. I had
to travel with the Eye Doctor to the villages where there was a
group of women prepared to work on improving health, or where
we wanted to start a new group.

At that time the doctor herself was talking to the people – partly in
vernacular, partly in English – and I had to translate for her. This
was to teach us how to give health education on trachoma. But
sometimes I could not quite say it the way she did. When I said
something different from what she said, I used to watch her to see
if she realised it, and when she didn't notice it, I went on in the
way I thought was right. She might say, 'This child has trachoma
because her face is not washed.' This was saying it too directly. I
had to go by a more roundabout way, and say, 'Trachoma is there
where it is too hot and where there is not enough water, and where
there are many flies. So you can sometimes catch the disease.' In
this way the person does not feel blamed. I had to put things my
way in order to keep the good relationship between the people and
myself. I did not tell the doctor that it would hurt if she said things
straightforwardly like that. I was still afraid that she could get
cross and I would lose my job.

Soon, the Eye Doctor no longer visited the groups each and every
time, and I went with one of the ophthalmic nursing students.
People who had been at the eye hospital already knew them, which
made it easier for us. After this group of students had finished
their training and left the eye department, I went alone with the
driver from the hospital.

After some months, when the groups were better organised, we
looked for a name for them and called them 'Care Groups'. A male
social worker joined us, and from then on we were known as 'Care
Group Motivators'. Many new groups were formed, and we had to
travel long distances on very bad roads. This made it difficult for
me when I was pregnant with my fifth child, a boy. I always say he

is a child of the Care Groups, because he saw all these places even before he was born.

'The nurses did not know what I was doing'

In the beginning I did not like to work with the Care Groups. When the Eye Doctor chose me to go out into the community, I did not understand why I should go. I found it was a big thing I could not manage. I even thought these people organising the project were not telling me the truth, they just wanted to get rid of me in the eye hospital. The thing which made it worse was, that from 7 o'clock in the morning I was supposed to start in the ward and do the daily duties. And when I had finished with that it would be 10 o'clock, and the others went for tea, but we had to go with the car. In the evenings we used to return late, but I still had to go to the hospital to report to the nurse on duty, as this was the rule at the hospital. The day nurses were already gone, it was the night nurses, and they knew nothing about why I should report. By then it was too late for the transport for hospital staff, and I had to walk home when it was dark. When I complained, I was told that I was rude. This hurt me and contributed to my feeling that this was a way to reject me.

The nurses did not know what I was doing. They thought I had to do health education and write a report. They did not understand how I could go alone into the community, as I did not give any treatment. What was I doing? Why should a nursing assistant go alone?

If there had been someone to encourage me and say, 'OK, you don't need to come to the ward when you come home late' it would have been better. At that time, I could not talk to the doctor about it, because I was still afraid of her, and we were trained not to say these things to our superiors. The nursing system reinforces our own traditional culture, where a young person will not correct an elderly person, even if she is wrong.

It made things very difficult for me that what I did in the community was not recognised by my superiors. Often I had no transport to go out, because it was being used by the doctors going to a clinic. This meant that people were thinking that only work done by doctors is important, and that what I was doing was not worthwhile. But doctors and community workers should work together, because both are important. Later, when a social worker had joined the project, we did have our own car, which made it easier.

However, the misunderstandings continued. The people in the hospital could not see why we should work till late in the evening. They did not understand that we could only have meetings in the community at a time which was suitable for the people. The women attending the Care Group meetings had their own work to do. They had to do the cooking and see that the children ate when they came back from school. It was only after the children had eaten that the mothers were free to go to a meeting. And I could not go away before finishing our discussion with the women. Later, the groups started to do practical things, like building mud stoves. You cannot manage to finish a mud stove in one hour! Or if you are sewing a 'wonder box' and finish only halfway, you will have to come back and start again in two weeks' time. Then people lose interest.

I am sad that even today, after more than 25 years of Care Groups, there are still many nurses in the hospital who do not know what Care Groups are. When people ask nurses, 'What is a Care Group Motivator?' some don't know at all. Others think they are the teachers of the Care Groups and put the desks in a row and then start teaching. Really! The word 'teach' is still very much in people's minds. They don't know that when we are out there we even go home visiting; we mix with people; we discuss things with them. There are only a few nurses who know from their mothers who are Care Group members that we are going to the villages to discuss health or other community problems with the people.

3. Learning on the job

'People wouldn't listen to my lessons'

When we started our work in the community we were not trained for the job. We were just pushed into the community and did not know what to do. I had to learn everything by myself while working with the people. It was an important experience which might be useful to others who are starting a project. When we visited the villages, it was my task to explain trachoma to the people and motivate them to act on its prevention. I started by teaching as I was used to doing in the hospital. Patients come to the hospital because they are sick. We give them health education because they happen to be there. We don't ask them whether they like it or not, or what they want to hear. We tell them what we think they should know. This is the way it is done in the hospital.

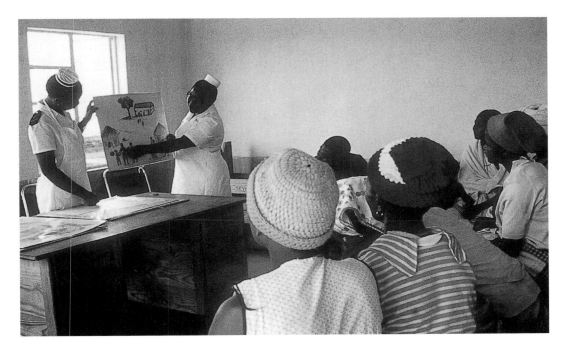

'I started by teaching as I was used to doing in the hospital.'
(Photo: E. Sutter)

But in the community it was different. The people were not interested in my lessons, and I was frustrated. I just told them what to do. It was not very effective. When I asked them questions they used to answer 'Yes, yes', or 'No, no'. We were too much in a hurry and wanted to get things moving. And the Eye Doctor wanted to hear a report that things went all right.

The Eye Doctor gave me books to read, but they didn't help me. She thought that it would be nice for me to read about health care in different countries. She did not realise that I could not read English very well (when I was in school , primary education was in the vernacular), so I read with little understanding. I couldn't say 'No' to her, and I did try to read what she had given me, but I had difficulties. Speaking is easier than reading and writing, because you choose the words you know. In the books there were always words I didn't know, and I couldn't guess or think what the words could mean. If it were today I would simply tell the doctor, 'I am not going to read all this.' But at that time I could not answer back, I just said 'Yes, yes, yes'.

Some things could have been helpful for us, but I didn't find a way of passing them on. I tried to read the books to the people and translate, which was not the correct thing. Then I asked some nurses to help me, and they said it would be easier if they would write something for me which I could read to the people. So I did this, and I was surprised to see that people still did not listen to me. The same happened with notes the doctor had written for us in order to prepare ourselves on what to tell the groups. We were just reading her notes to the groups, and nobody could understand what we were reading, and the people were sleeping.

I was always thinking, 'Why are the women doing that? What must I do?' I was thinking all night what I should do and how I could talk to the people so that they would listen. I was so frustrated. I used to cry. It was too difficult for me to work in the community.

4. Making friends and building trust

'I changed my method of doing things': stories from the old ladies

At last I decided to change my method of doing things. I started to visit homes, to sit down and relax and talk with the people, introducing myself in order to make friends with them until they were used to me. In this way I got the stories from the old ladies. I had already heard some stories from the old people when I worked in the eye department in the wards, and I got more stories out in the community.

As I was supposed to work with the groups I felt quite guilty when I went to talk to people at their homes instead of meeting with the group. Nobody told me to do that. It was my own secret, and I did not tell the nurses or the Eye Doctor. My superiors would have thought I was just wasting time, not even talking about health when visiting homes. But I got a lot of information from the people when talking generally with them about social issues. I was sharing my difficulties with them, and they gave me advice and were happy that I also had the same problems they had, and that we were the same. In this way they started trusting me. Sometimes they started talking about health, and they were ready to listen to me, because it was their own problem and they knew what we were talking about.

It was the same with the Care Group members. When we were sitting together, maybe waiting for the others to arrive for a meeting, someone could make a remark about some difficulties she had in her family, and I could say, 'I am also faced with that.' Then the people felt free to talk about their own problems.

All this took a long time and I gained a lot of experience. The main thing was that now we trusted each other. Now people knew why we were there. I learned how to approach the community and to understand the culture. I think this was the correct way for me to learn, because then I began to fit in with the people.

I learned most from the grandmothers: the way to be respectful; the way to approach the elderly, and not to look down at their customs. Then I realised that it is important to sit down with the people and to discuss instead of giving lessons. I learned that just to give lots of advice and tell people what to do does not help people. Instead of encouraging them, it makes them feel ignorant.

Since those days, I have also learned new ways of teaching. People understand and remember better when I use group discussions, pictures, songs, drawings and role play. By discussing together they find their own solutions to their problems. At the end they will be able to say, 'This was our own idea!' Then it is something people want to do, and they will do it well, unlike when they are told to do something that they do not understand. Now, when people are stuck during a discussion I quickly invent a story that could help them to find a solution to their problem. Sometimes when the group cannot find a solution I just say the opposite of what should be done and ask them many questions. Then they will think hard and see that this is not good and they will find the best way of solving it.

'When I started listening to the people, I learned many things'

People have very good ideas in many cases. From the elderly I learned about what they do in cases of measles, or when they are sick. For example, a child with measles is isolated and given milk to drink. They may put something in the eyes, which can be wrong, but this we can change. When I find out from people how they used to do things traditionally, I never blame them for doing something wrong. I always first praise them for the good things they do. This makes them happy and they see that we respect them, and it creates a calm atmosphere. After this I can carefully correct the dangerous things they may do by replacing them with something useful.

I learned that when we discussed things, it was best to start with what I had heard in the community. People like to have their own methods discussed, in order to know which of their remedies is good and which could be dangerous. When starting on a subject like measles, I asked the group first what they knew about measles. First they said they knew nothing. But when I told them the stories about measles I had heard from the old ladies, they looked at each other and were surprised how I could know this. Then they started telling what they knew and from there it was easy to discuss. In this way I managed to build on all they knew and carefully added what they didn't know. Not rushing, but very carefully.

'I managed to build on all they knew'

It worked very well when we were talking about the new type of soft porridge for the children. It was not a lecture, it was a discussion and finding out from the elderly people, and they were telling us their story. One old lady started, 'You know, these young mothers, they don't want to listen. We tell them how things were done in olden times. They think it's over, it's not for them.' Then we asked the young mothers how they were giving the soft porridge. They said that they were cooking the porridge in the big pot where they cook for the family, and then they would take part of it and save it for the child, maybe just adding some sugar. But the elderly people were against this way of doing things. Then we asked what method the elderly people had used. They told us that they collected a special root which they boiled and made juice of it and added it to the porridge. This was better than plain porridge with water only.

From what the old people told us I got an idea. I was thinking, 'What must I do with that?' I praised the old ladies, and said they were right, and they were very happy. We asked them if they could still manage to find these roots to put in the children's porridge, and they said, 'No, not now. We used to stay along the river where the trees are growing, and we could manage to get the roots easily. But now we are not near the rivers. We were taken off the place where we stayed. We can't get the roots any more.' We asked what they could take instead of these roots, and they said, 'There is nothing, and that is why the young ones are cooking as they do now.'

This was my starting point for something new in my work with the groups. I said, 'There is something to replace that. The peanuts are from under the ground like roots. You can dry peanuts, pound them and use them for the porridge.' Then we agreed that at the following meeting we would cook the porridge adding peanuts. We pounded the peanuts in the home of one of the mothers, and we made weaning porridge with half maize flour and half peanuts. They tasted it and found that it tasted nice. After that they accepted it. We were careful not to blame the young mothers for doing something wrong. If the elderly people understand and accept it, the young ones will be free to change to the new porridge. That is why it worked with the young mothers. Now when the elderly have some peanuts they give them to the grandchildren.

From the porridge with peanuts the discussion went further about other things one could add, like vegetables or eggs. 'Oh, eggs? Do children eat eggs?' they said. I said, 'Yes, they make the children grow strong. I don't know, but you may know why children should not eat eggs.' They told me that in old times eggs were taboo for girls and women to eat, because they believed that when labour is difficult there is an egg in the way. I finally did manage to convince the elderly people that children should eat eggs. I explained that there are many things about which we do not really know whether they are good or not. We think girls should not eat eggs. But there are many cultures where children do get eggs, and these children are healthy and grow well. The elderly people believed me because they trusted me, and therefore felt that what I said was right. This is the most important thing for people; to trust. If they don't trust somebody he or she can say things that are good and useful, but people will not accept them. But I realised that for things that have to do with culture I must be very careful and find the correct way to discourage something that is not good. All the time, I was learning more and more from the people, and I could compare what I knew from reading, or from the doctors, with what the community knew. To me, the community is a good teacher.

'When people know, they will act'

When people are not aware of a problem and of what causes it, they will not do anything about it. But when they know, they will act. For example people thought flies are caused by milk. Now they know that it is not milk but cow dung that attracts them, and they know what to do. They also did not know that flies on the eyes spread diseases. Now with knowledge they act on it. People have realised that flies do not come when the face is clean. It does not need much water to wash the face. But when one is not aware that it is important, one does not wash frequently, even when there is enough water. Now with awareness people use the little water they have according to priorities. Also mothers of malnourished children don't see why they should get health education when they are coming for the first time to the nutrition unit. But when we discuss with the mothers, individually and in groups, they can find out for themselves at which point things started to go wrong with their child. Then they become interested and are willing to learn, and they come back every week and want to know more.

'Health education works well in small gatherings'

For health education, groups should be small, like the Care Groups. The members have become friends and they help each other to implement what they have learned. Then the neighbours see what is happening in the Care Group's homes, and when it looks good they want to imitate. When something is beautiful, for example a well-decorated wall, all adopt it and want to do the same. The same is true for good hygiene, because the house and people look beautiful. This is why I like to work with the Care Groups, where we can discuss and where people feel free to talk.

When discussing with small groups it is easier to observe the people and see how they react to what you are saying. Sometimes it can happen that I see one member gets disturbed while we are talking about a certain disease. Then I know that she might have the problem we are talking about and I continue my talk differently.

I will not ask the mother the same day why she was worried, but I ask her next time how she liked the discussion. It is important that we always observe well in order not to hurt people. And we must always be ready to adapt ourselves and change to another topic if necessary.

I have observed many times that health education given to great gatherings, which are without commitment, has little effect. Changing knowledge into practice does not work without personal motivation. If we want health education to be successful it needs enough time for motivation. Some of our superiors do not understand this.

Let me take an example. People are usually cooking vegetables for a very long time. If I want them to change and cook the vegetables for a short time, on a house visit I taste the vegetables the mother has cooked for a long time and I even praise her. I tell her it tastes nice and ask her how she cooked them. Then I will tell her that there are many ways to cook vegetables. And she will ask, 'How do you cook them?' So I ask her if she wants me to come to her home so we can do it together. We cook the vegetables together and she tastes the result. Then I can explain why I cook these vegetables for a few minutes only. I do not tell her she is wrong. She is going to think for herself. Next time in the group when we talk about cooking food she will come with the new method. We are also cooking in the group together. Many times we have cooked under the tree in the shade. The women use their own pots, not my pots, and they bring the wood. So, let's say there are not so many, maybe 5 or 6 members; we cook these vegetables together, and I explain to them. And next time, there may be a big group, but I am not going to do it myself. They are going to do it for the big group. So I think it needs both, working with individuals on house visits, and working in groups. It takes a long time, but people will then really do the correct thing, not only say, 'Yes, yes', and not do it.

5. Formal training at last – and a journey to England

The starting period in my work as a Care Group Motivator was really very difficult. The worst thing was that it took two years until I got the chance to attend a training course. Then I was sent for three months to a training centre for health advisors where I learned about nutrition and health education. After that I could go for many more short courses, for example on leadership training, food production, deep trench vegetable growing, child development and many more. After I had been with the Care Groups for ten years, I was sent to England for one year's training in Primary Health Care and Community Development at Manchester University, and in Child Nutrition in London.

My journey to England

I did not know what happens when you fly in an aeroplane. I was scared. I thought for flying you need trousers which are tied fast at the bottom – and I had no trousers. When I got to the airport, I did not see men in trousers tied at the bottom. People were dressed normally. Some people waiting in the waiting hall were nervous, others were relaxed. So I thought, it can't be so bad, and I relaxed. When the call came for boarding, I was careful not to be in front nor in the back of the queue, so that I could see how it went, and that still some people had to come after me. I thought there is very little room in the plane, but when I got in, it was so beautiful, with beautiful seats. So I sat down, relieved, but fearing how it will be on take-off. When it took off, most people closed their eyes. Were they afraid to see what happens? But I wanted to see exactly what is happening. So it took off, steep into the sky, and I felt OK. At Nairobi the plane went down, zzzzzz..., and then up again. At Amsterdam down, and up again. By the time we went down in Zürich I was used to it.

I spent two weeks with the Eye Doctor in Switzerland, and then came the flight to London. To change the plane at Heathrow we had to take our luggage and walk through long passages. The change to the Manchester flight was terrible. At the exit there was no plane, but a small bus. They said I must get into the bus. I said, 'No, I can't go into the bus. I go by plane to Manchester, not by bus.' I refused again, but finally I had to give in. I thought, let me wait and see what is going to happen. The bus went round many corners, and then stopped in front of a plane. Then it was better.

At Manchester airport most people were fetched by someone, but nobody came for me. I thought, 'I must be careful not to be cheated – but I do have to take a taxi to the hostel.' I went to a taxi, but the driver did not wait till the taxi was full, the way they do at home. He drove with me alone. 'So I am being cheated', I thought. But then I saw that other taxis also only had one or two persons. When we came to the hostel, the taxi left me there. There was nobody around. I knocked at all the doors, but nobody was answering. I was the first one to arrive. By and by other students arrived. Only then did I learn that you don't knock at the door, but you have to press a button for the bell.

The doctors found a good person who paid for the training, but she was not with me to introduce me to Manchester. I had to find out everything by myself: how to live in a town in England, how the buses function, what happens at university – everything. It was difficult in the beginning, but at the end I knew better than the other students who had been mothered all the time by some organisation. I had to study very hard, learning how to read books and how to write essays. But I managed, and gained a lot. I made many good friends who came from all over the world, and I could share ideas with them. In time, I started to enjoy my studies, and the lecturers were happy with me. The course was a good thing for the Care Groups, as I learned much that was useful for the community. I now have more to offer to the groups. There is still much to learn, and I am still attending courses and workshops, some even in other countries, like Kenya.

6. Summing up: I like the work in the community – but I also have problems

Care Groups are now more than 25 years old, and since they started I have never stopped working in the Project. Apart from all the good things I enjoyed in this job there were two issues which worried me then, and still worry me now: the lack of a career structure for nursing assistants, and combining the job with looking after my family.

After the first medical superintendent left, the hospital management took very little interest in the Care Groups for many years. This has changed recently, but for a long time they did not realise what type of work we were doing. One result of this was that except that I advanced from Motivator to Senior Motivator, I was never given any promotion or a salary increase for my work. Many times I felt like leaving the Care Groups to go back to the wards, working again as an assistant nurse. It would have been an easier job, with regular working hours and more free time to be with my children. But I could not do that to my people in the community. They counted on me. So I kept on struggling.

Now I like being a Care Group Motivator, and I don't feel any more that I was allocated to the Care Groups in order to get rid of me in the eye hospital. I have realised that I was sent to work with the community because the doctor trusted me. But it also meant that there was very little space left for my own personal life.

For most of the years when I was working with the Care Groups and attending all these courses my five children were still living at home. It was difficult because I was away from home too much. I am worried that I have not been a good mother for my children. They suffered because I did not have enough time for them. I am happy that they don't complain – and they are even proud of what I do.

Chapter 2

The growing Care Groups; the first 8 years

Dzovo va tlhuvutsa ehubyeni

The hides become well softened while you attend the court

While sitting and listening to lengthy court procedures, the men often occupy themselves by kneading hides to soften them (a procedure that takes a long time). While they sit there they listen and learn a lot.

Chapter 2

The growing Care Groups; the first 8 years

1. The founding of the first groups

The Care Group Project was started because of the problem of trachoma in the area. The idea of health groups in the community was new to everybody. People had to be informed before anything could be started. The first step was to talk with the chiefs and other key people in the three pilot communities and to get their co-operation. In the beginning I was scared to go to the chiefs because in our culture a woman is not supposed to do that. But when I went to the villages with our social worker, he taught me how to talk with them. He succeeded in making the chiefs accept that a woman was allowed to speak to them. The chiefs were scared we would do family planning, which men don't like. The social worker explained what we were doing, and then the chiefs accepted.

The chiefs were then asked to call for a village meeting to discuss trachoma, to explain the functioning of the Project and enrol voluntary helpers. To prepare for the enrolment I used to visit the place beforehand several times and make some friends in the community who were willing to help. When at the end of the village function volunteers were invited to give their names, my friends were the first to come forward. This encouraged others to join as well. It was made very clear from the start that the groups were voluntary, and helpers would not be paid.

'We changed to normal dresses'

When we went to the families to prepare for a village meeting many people did not understand why we came. The Care Groups were the first organisation where people from the hospital went out into the community to talk about health. People used to hear about health when they went to the clinic, but there were no people who went to the houses to give health education. Once an old man

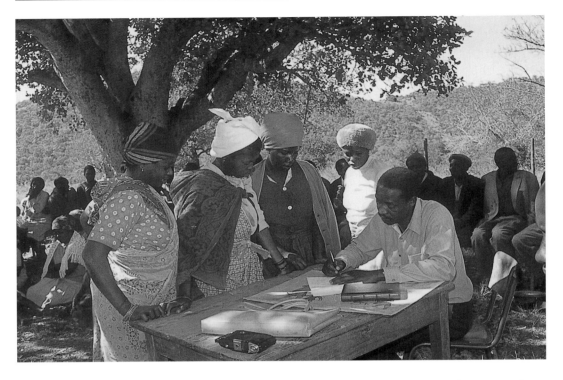

The founding of one of the first Care Groups. At a village gathering volunteers give their names to Care Group Motivator Andrew Radebe. (Photo: E. Sutter)

chased me with a stick, shouting, 'You have now finished killing the people in the hospital, and now you are starting to hunt for us here in the community! When we are sick we know where to go!' At that time I was still wearing the white uniform from the hospital. People were not used to seeing nurses in the village. It happened often that people in the community were afraid of doctors and nurses, especially if rumours went round about vaccination campaigns in schools, and they were made to believe that the injection was killing the children. Then the children were running away when they saw a car coming with people in white uniforms. As long as people took us for nurses, it was often difficult to visit a family, because when a child saw us, it just cried, and we couldn't discuss with the mother. We couldn't stay in that family long enough to talk.

For this reason we changed later to normal dresses, which were blue. We had a lot of discussions before we were allowed to do this, because the regulations said nursing staff must always wear white. The blue dresses made a great difference. We could now go to the homes and play with the children, and everybody was free and relaxed. Then people found out what we were trying to do, and they started to think that we were good people to work with.

Attacking trachoma: 'Blindness is not a heritage'

When the groups met for the first time, we explained first of all about trachoma; that the eyes are itchy and feel as though they have sand in them. In children the eyes are often discharging, and older people also get red and watery eyes. The disease is infectious.

I then asked the members if they knew such a disease and if there was a name for it in their own language, Tsonga. People started discussing and told me that many people had this disease. They called it *mavoni*. All their children had it when they were still young, and people believed that if children did not have discharging eyes early in life they would not be able to see well by the time they started school. In fact, people had observed correctly that after the first infection in early childhood the disease gets better on its own, and the children can see well again. Later, when the women in the Care Groups knew more about trachoma, they could convince people that *mavoni* was not a good thing for their children. There are other beliefs about trachoma: a woman who does not tell her mother-in-law when she is pregnant with another child will get sore eyes, and the old lady will get *shinyeku*, which means in-turning eyelashes.

This was a good platform for me to start from, as the Eye Doctor had told me that trachoma has different stages. I said, 'Yes, we are talking about the same disease.' I explained more about trachoma and why it causes blindness and asked what they were doing for this disease. They said, 'We put some traditional medicine, but it does not help. When it is severe some people go to the hospital. We have no other ways. There is no clinic here. And we have no transport and no money to pay at the hospital.' From there we could start a discussion on the prevention of trachoma. I asked the Care Group members if they knew that they could prevent this disease, and that this would save them from going to the hospital. 'How?', they asked.

I explained that trachoma will not come to them if they wash their face and hands frequently, each one using their own face cloth. 'That is impossible', they said. 'We only have two face cloths in the family, one for the husband, and nobody has to touch it, and one for the mother who shares it with all the children.'

I told them that when we were still children, we used to wash ourselves with our hands. They said, 'Our husbands have seen the face cloths in Johannesburg and brought them from there, which made us think that face cloths are more civilised.'

I answered, 'It is not bad to use face cloths, but if you use only one cloth for the family the cloth will spread trachoma from one person to the others. We could make cloths for every family member from a good piece of old cloth, and decorate each with a different colour, one for every child.'

I went on to explain, 'Another thing which makes trachoma worse is having flies around. Flies lay their eggs in dirty wet places. We can chase the flies away by cleanliness of our bodies and surroundings. Instead of a rubbish heap where the flies are multiplying we can dig a rubbish pit where we can cover the dirt with soil, and when the pit is full we can plant a fruit tree.'

'If we can practice all this and give advice to everybody in the community, then we will only need eye ointment for those who are affected. Then people will not get blind from trachoma. As we say in Tsonga, "Blindness is not a heritage".'

The women go into action

We kept on discussing until the women said, 'You can show us what trachoma looks like and then we can do the treatment. If you can give us the ointment, we can put it in our children's eyes.'

I asked, 'What about the neighbours? We told you that this is an infectious disease. If you give the ointment to your child only, and if, after your tube is finished, your child is going to play with other children who have trachoma, your child will get trachoma again. Children like each other. When playing they touch each other. And the flies are there also. They go to the eyes, and the children get infected again. What are you going to do? Will you keep your children at home after you put ointment in? Should they no more play with other children?' They said, 'Ooooh! That is not possible!'

'So what are you going to do?' I asked. They said, 'You had better give us enough ointment, so that we can give it also to the other families.'

We made a list of those who wanted to learn and made an appointment for the next meeting. We taught them how to examine eyes for trachoma and apply the ointment. We also taught them to keep notes on the number of tubes they used. We went to work on arithmetic together several times, using stones, working out how many tubes are needed when two people in one family were using one tube together. And when we went through their notebooks with them, they could tell us exactly how many tubes of eye ointment were needed.

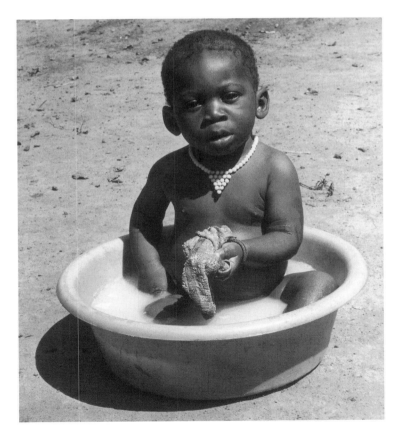

A face-cloth for every member of the family. (Photo: E. Sutter)

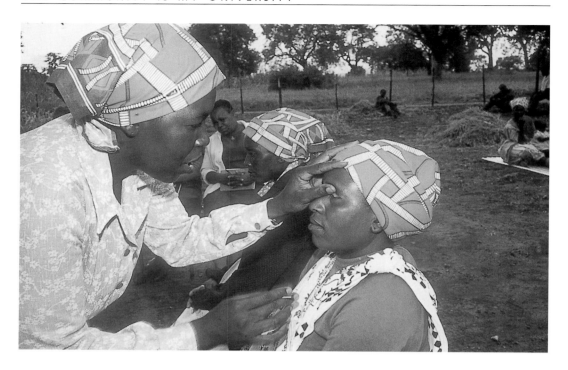

'We taught the Care Group members how to examine eyes for trachoma.'
(Photo: E. Sutter)

There were a few problems with some members who were keeping
the ointment for themselves and were only giving it to their friends
or relatives. We discovered what was happening when the children
kept on having eye diseases and never got better. We reminded the
women of what we had discussed before about prevention and
treatment. How could the others trust a Care Group member who
was keeping the ointment for herself? When people went to her
and asked for ointment for their children, and she said she had
none, and yet people could see ointment in her children's eyes,
how could they trust her? Many women wanted to give ointment to
relatives staying far away, but in the end they understood that it
would be useless, because if only one family is treated the
children will get infected again.

The Care Groups develop their own ways of doing things

In the beginning, the Eye Doctor had thought that health workers from the hospital would examine school children for trachoma. The Care Group members would then visit the children who had trachoma in their homes, because when a child has trachoma, other family members are usually also infected. But the Care Groups didn't like this plan. As they had learned to examine eyes, they wanted to look for trachoma by themselves – and they did this most efficiently!

The original plan was that each Care Group member would take care of about 10 families, and go to them to give them health education and ointment. However, when the Care Group members went visiting homes as individuals they often experienced difficulties. People said, 'What can you tell us? Where were you trained?' So they started to visit as a group.

We Motivators only discovered that the Care Groups had worked out their own method of visiting homes when we went to one of the villages to find out exactly how many families had trachoma. The group members said it was impossible to visit all the houses on the same day, as they had started to go as a group. I had thought it would not be possible for the whole group to visit one family, but they found it easy. First the whole group went dancing and singing through the streets, till they found a place in the shade where they beat drums and danced. The people came flocking, and the group told them about what they had learned from the Motivators. After that, they started visiting the homes in smaller groups, supporting each other. When they arrived at the houses they did not start by telling what they had come for. They were just singing and dancing, and people would come from other homes. Then they started with health education, and the people liked it. They invited them to ask questions and bring their children for eye ointment. Then they would teach the mothers how to apply ointment.

In this way they could show the community that they know some-thing about health. From then on it was easier to go into the houses and to give ointment. And when the people discovered that Care Group members even knew how to evert eye lids in order to examine for trachoma, and that they could teach something and apply ointment, they said, 'The nurses are coming!', and the members were proud of that. By that time the members were strong enough to go visiting on their own, and each one started to take care of ten families in her street.

'Many people were happy with Care Groups ... but not everybody'

Many people in the community were happy with the Care Groups from the beginning, and respected them, but not everybody. Some found it difficult to see their purpose and could not understand why people were leaving the hospital to come into their communities. They said, 'No, there must be something behind this. Using petrol to come here in a car, just to say "Hello", to prevent a disease, that is not possible.'

Many people could not see what face cloths or rubbish pits could have to do with good health for their families. When the young mothers wanted to make a rubbish pit, some old ladies were refusing. They said, 'You are now even making a grave to bury us.' They didn't understand what it was. But when they saw that it was better to throw all the rubbish there, and the surroundings were clean, and at the end they could plant a fruit tree in the pit, they started to see the sense of it.

Another thing was that some people thought that the hospital was now right in their community, and that they were going to get free treatment. They came when they saw us and started to complain about their stomachs and such things, and wanted medicine, and were disappointed that they did not get treatment or an injection, but only talk. People thought we were carrying injections around, and when we saw a patient, we could just inject them.

When we stopped giving eye ointment, because the hospital had no money any more, and we were always talking about how personal hygiene would help, some people were discouraged and said, 'Oh, we don't get ointment, so what is the use of going to Care Groups?' But after some time they realised at last that other things were important too. It gave people courage to see how their homes improved, and to know that they were doing it for the health of their families. People began to see that what the Care Groups were doing was good. The schoolteachers praised them because the children were coming to school clean and with no trachoma.

'Work means money': working without payment?

Care Group members have always been volunteers, and work for the sake of their families and their community with no pay. This has not usually caused problems. But one day it happened that somebody asked a group, 'How much are you earning if you keep on going there? You say they are teaching you how to see trachoma in somebody's eyes, and you keep on looking into people's eyes, and then they give you ointment to treat. Are they giving you money?' They said, 'No'.

The response was, 'You are very stupid! Those people from the hospital are earning money. They are just cheating you when they come here and you keep on following them. You are helping them to do their work. They think you have to go and do things for them.' Then these members came back to us and said that they wanted to be paid. I was shivering when I heard this. I started to sweat. I didn't know what to do. I had no money to pay them.

At that time the Care Group was meeting under the tree next to the shop. This gave me the idea for a story which was different from eyes or ointment – one about a shopkeeper:

'There was a woman who was married to a very good husband, and they had 5 children. The husband went to Johannesburg to work, and the mother remained at home with the children. Suddenly he stopped sending money home because he got another wife in Johannesburg. The wife kept going to the shop, asking for mealie meal, and promised the husband would send money to pay for it. The shopkeeper kept on giving her mealie meal until he discovered that it would never be paid for. So he stopped. Then that lady was going around to other people asking for mealie meal. They were giving it to her until they were tired, then they also stopped. She was not working, she was staying at home with the children. So the children were starving. They kept on crying.

'Then one day the shopkeeper was walking around and found that the lady was just lying under the tree, and the children were crying and very weak. So he was afraid that these people were dying of hunger. He went to the shop and took a full bag of mealie meal and took it to that lady. He told her that she should quickly cook for the children, so that they would stop crying. The woman got up to cook for the children, and the children had their food. They were now happy, and playing again. The lady went to the shop and told the shopkeeper, "You told me to cook for the children. Now that I have finished cooking, will you please pay me?"'

When they heard the story the Care Group women all laughed, 'She was a stupid lady!' Then I said, 'You told us that you have a problem, and we are trying to solve that problem with you. We have promised to give you ointment. We offer to come with the hospital car, which is using money for petrol. We have contributed towards solving your problems. We are also going to share the knowledge we have with you. The only thing you have to do is to take the ointment and go around and treat your own people. Where will the money for paying you come from?' 'Ah yes,' they said, 'you are right!' Then I said, 'No, I don't mean you must say I am right. I think it is very difficult for you to do that. So the ointment I am giving you today will be the last. I am not going to bring more ointment. I am now moving to another group to help them as I was helping you.' Then they said, 'Who said we wanted to be paid? Nobody wanted to be paid!' So the solution just came on its own and the women were happy again to volunteer without payment.

As this story worked well with that group, I have used it many times since then. Sometimes you find that a person who does not think carefully will just follow the advice of outsiders, and start to demand money. A good story makes the women think hard, and they themselves can find the answer to their question.

These people who disturb the Care Group members by making them feel they are being exploited are often people from outside who do not understand how the groups work. They do not have problems with money themselves – they can just take a bus to go to the hospital when they are sick. But the Care Group member has no money to go to the hospital when her child has trachoma or diarrhoea or when it is malnourished. She could prevent these diseases with the knowledge she gets from the Care Group. The problem is that in our culture we do care for our relatives – but for others, people don't want to volunteer. Nowadays it is like this, that when you do something for somebody you want to be paid. The relationship to work is money.

2. The movement expands

The home visits often motivated other people in the community to join the Care Group. Community members who were not present at the mass meeting when Care Groups were introduced learned about what the groups were doing when they went visiting homes. In the evening, when a Care Group member finished work and went to visit one of her 10 families, when she got there she might find people from two other families already there, and others might join them. So she would have a good time discussing with them what we had done with the Care Group in the last meeting. Sometimes after such a discussion somebody from one of these families would decide to join the Care Group, and then the new member would take another ten families.

A community starts a new Care Group

There was one community where many people had friends or relatives in the place where one of the first three groups was. When they visited each other they heard about the Care Groups, and when they went back to their community they were talking about it. So the men said, 'We have to stop this. The people from the hospital should not just pass through here, they should stop here.' We were called to the Tribal Office. There they told us that they heard that we had started a clinic at that other place and were treating people. We said, 'That's not true. We are not treating people. People are treating themselves.' And we explained what we do, and they said that they also wanted something like that. We said, 'That's fine, you remain discussing amongst yourselves and think about how you want to do it.' They said they would write us a letter, but in the end we just got a message to tell us the date to start. When we arrived at the Tribal Office, we found that there were so many people. We explained to them what Care Groups do, and some of them volunteered. That's how that Care Group started.

People liked the Care Groups very much. When we started there were three groups, and by the end of the first year the number of groups in our area was 27. Only a few groups were started by the Project Team. Most groups got started on their own, and then called us to assist. There were also Care Groups which were starting other groups. After a group had started to treat trachoma, a neighbouring place might call the members of that group to come and tell them how they started it. After that they started their own group in their community, and when they were ready, they called us to help them. When we reached there we often found the group already organised, having chosen their chairlady. Some groups even thought of going to neighbouring places specially to show them what they had learned. For example the members of one Care Group went to another community to demonstrate how to build a mud stove.

3. The groups start new activities

In some of the villages that started Care Groups, trachoma was not a major concern; the women were more worried about typhoid or bilharzia, and we adapted the programme to their needs. In the groups that were busy with trachoma prevention, the mothers also wanted to know about other health problems, especially those affecting their children, like measles and malnutrition. Over the years, the groups became active in many different ways. Not only the members but the Motivators learned many things.

Healthy children

We showed the Care Group members how they could see if their child was growing well, and told them about the type of food children need. They learned how to read the 'Road to Health' chart and were encouraged to attend the child health clinic regularly. When they looked at the chart and saw the weight of the child dropping, they could think of what was happening to the child at that time. They might remember that it had severe diarrhoea or some other problem. Then the mothers were motivated to learn how to prepare the oral rehydration fluid and how to prevent diarrhoea. Another activity which was important for the prevention of malnutrition was the cooking of a good weaning food, as powdered milk was too expensive. We cooked a mixture of maize meal and finely ground peanuts. This tastes nice and the children like it.

Gardens for a better diet

It is very important to add green vegetables or yellow fruit to the children's porridge to prevent vitamin A deficiency and childhood blindness. When we discussed this, the Care Group members became interested in how to produce vegetables and fruit. As we had not enough skills in vegetable growing, I was sent together with a co-worker to the Valley Trust, where they teach people about how to grow food in a dry area like ours (see Appendix p. 265).

The Valley Trust and Deep Trench Gardening: a doctor who wouldn't take 'No' for an answer

The Valley of a Thousand Hills is not far from South Africa's east coast in the Province Kwazulu Natal. The valley used to be barren as a result of over-grazing, and its people were poor and malnourished. The doctor in the valley's health centre became more and more frustrated by his powerlessness in the face of rampant malnutrition, but when he asked a professor of agriculture at Durban University for advice on food production in the valley the answer was a categorical, 'Impossible, on this soil you'll never produce anything.'

The doctor did not accept the verdict, and advertised for agricultural extension officers. Fifty replied. The doctor chose the most infertile patch in the area, and told the applicants that the one who could grow vegetables there within one year, without fertiliser or irrigation, would get the job. One of them said, 'I can do it. I will take the valley on the hill.' He cut the grass and dug a trench 1m x 2m in area (the size of a vegetable bed) and 1m deep, setting the topsoil aside. Then he filled the trench with alternate layers of grass and organic domestic refuse, 30 cm deep, and about 10 cm of subsoil. Finally he replaced the topsoil. First a leguminous crop was planted, and dug in at the flowering stage. After that he planted the vegetables.

This is the method that has since been taught by the Valley Trust. Except for the first week the young plants do not require any watering. After that, in Natal the dew of the night is sufficient, and even in arid areas like the Northern Province watering is only necessary every two weeks.

Today the Valley of a Thousand Hills is one big vegetable growing area. People have enough food, there is no more malnutrition, and the people have an income from selling the surplus crops. The Health Centre is now a training institution for agricultural development.

When we returned home we showed the groups what we had learned, demonstrating the method. The Care Group members started home gardens where they produced beautiful vegetables, and they could feed their families without buying vegetables. They shared their knowledge with their neighbours, and many families started gardens. The community was happy with what the Care Group members taught them. From 1980 there was a very severe drought for many years. It was very interesting to see in the third year of drought, that the Care Group members who were digging the trench deep enough still had beautiful green vegetables, while others, who were still using the traditional method of hoeing only, had nothing growing.

Communal gardens – and a revolving loan scheme

When we visited the homes to look at the gardens we found that many families were worried that the goats and the chickens were destroying their nice plots, as the gardens were not properly fenced. The Care Group members asked me what they could do to protect their vegetables. I told them that this was for the group to discuss. In one village, the members came up with the idea of asking the village chief for a big plot where each member would be allocated a piece large enough for the needs of the family, so that they could be away from the chickens and goats. The chief offered a field where they could cut thorn trees to fence their garden. But before they started to plough the garden the Tribal Office fined them for cutting trees. The group members were worried, and they told us about the problem. The Care Group Project offered the group a revolving loan to buy fencing material, garden tools and seeds. The group organised a garden committee which looked after the running of the garden, and decided as a group how to pay the loan back to the project. For example the women went together as a group to work for other people in the fields or to collect wood for them. The money the group earned in this way was used to refund the revolving loan, and we were able to give a new loan to the next group wanting to start a garden.

Communal gardens have now become very popular. Almost every Care Group has a garden, and it is still the thing the Care Groups like most. The gardens benefit the community, as those who do not have the time to plant themselves can buy local fresh vegetables at a price they can afford.

Changes in Care Group activities 1976 – 1983

Year	Trachoma	Vegetable gardens	Child nutrition	ORF chlorin.	Mud stoves	Toilets	Bulk buying
	+					+	
1976	++		+			+	
	+++					++	
	+++		+			++	
	+++		+			++	
1977	+++	+	+			++	
	+++	+	+			++	
	+++	++				++	
	++++	++	+			++	
1978	++++	+++	+			++	
	++++	+++	+			+	
	+++++	+++	+			+	
	+++++	+++	+				
	++++++	+++	+				
1979	++++++	+++	+	+			
	++++++	++++	+	++			
	+++++	+++++	++	+++			
	+++	+++++	++	++++			
	++	+++++	++	++++			
1980	+	+++++	++	+++++			
	+	+++++	++	++++++			
	+	+++++	+++	++++++	+		
	+	+++++	+++	++++++	++		
	+	+++++	+++	++++++	++		
1981	+	+++++	++++	++++++	++		
	+	+++++	++++	++++++	+		
	+	++++	+++++	+++++	++		
	+	++++	+++++	++++	+		
	+	++++	+++++	+++	++		
1982	+	++++	+++++	++	++		
	+	++++	+++++	++	+++	+	+
	+	+++++	+++++	++	++	+	+
	+	+++++	+++++	++	+++	++	++
	+	+++++	+++++	+	+++	++	++
1983	+	+++++	+++++	+	+++	+++	+++
	+	+++++	+++++	+	++++	+++	+++
	+	+++++	+++++	+	++++	+++	+++
	+	+++++	+++++	+	++++	++	+++
	+	++++++	++++++	+	++++	+++	++++

Crosses represent the number of groups involved in a particular activity:

+ Little (or sporadic) activity in a few groups only

++++++ Main activity in almost all groups

Saving fuel

Another big problem in our area is to find wood for cooking. The women complained that they had to spend many hours collecting wood far away, and they had not enough time for other work and to look after the children. They were also often fined for cutting trees for firewood that were still green, or when they were in the wrong place. We introduced two methods to save fuel: 'wonder boxes' and mud stoves. (Solar cookers had not yet been introduced.) I learned to make wonder boxes from the Valley Trust, where I had also learned about deep trench gardening. Two cushion covers are sewn and filled with discarded polystyrene packing material, hay, peanut shells, or any other locally available insulating material. For cooking, the food only needs to be brought to the boil, and then the pot is put into the box between the two cushions. The mother can then go to work, and when the children come home from school they find their food ready to eat (pattern & instructions p. 266).

The idea of building mud stoves came from Botswana. One of our doctors had visited there and has seen a fuel-saving mud stove which was easy to build and was working well. We learned from him how to build these stoves and demonstrated them to the Care Groups. The stove can be built in one day, using mud bricks people make themselves. When the stove is used, the heat of the fire bakes the bricks. The women realised that when using the stove they were saving a lot of wood. Instead of going to collect wood nearly every day, it was now enough to go once or twice a week. A mud stove keeps the house warm in winter, there is always hot water ready, and the kitchen is free of smoke. Before, the houses were full of smoke, and when people went too near to the fire to warm themselves, many burn accidents used to happen. People like the stoves, and there are communities where there is now a stove in nearly every family (building method p. 268).

We tried a third way of solving the fuel problem, but that was less successful. The doctors told us about a tree called *Leucaena*, which is used in many countries for fuel-wood plantations. We thought it would be a good idea to try to grow these trees. In the first place where we made a trial the trees grew well and the people were happy. Then we encouraged the women in another place to plant the trees. They worked very hard and had great hopes. They thought they would never again have to go for wood. But the soil was too dry and there were too many termites, and the trees did not grow.

This was a good lesson for us. We did not yet have enough experience with the *Leucaena* tree, and we should have told the people that we were still finding out how the tree could be used and where it would grow best. People must know when something is still on trial, so that they will not have wrong expectations. Even in the place where the trees grew well, they still did not produce enough wood for fuel. Now we know that in our region *Leucaena* is not suitable for this purpose. But we did find out that the tree can be used in many other ways. People even call it the 'wonder tree'. It is fast-growing, and when it is cut it makes many new branches. The women use the branches to support their tomatoes, beans and peas. The leaves are good food for cattle and goats, and the tree fertilises the soil by making it richer in nitrogen. The tree is very valuable for communal gardens, and many groups are using these trees for the agroforestry method. They plant the trees around the garden, and in rows between the plots as a windbreak and to give them shade when they are working.

Oral rehydration and safe drinking water

During the early years of the Project there was a cholera epidemic in the region. We didn't see any cholera here, but still people quickly took it up as a problem, because people were talking about it. People were thinking, 'When it comes here, what will we do? How can we prevent it before it arrives?' They were therefore willing to learn about oral rehydration fluid and water purification. They even made a song about cholera, how you get it, and what to do about it.

We demonstrated a method of water purification, using 'Javel' (a chlorine-containing bleaching fluid). We told people to use 20 drops of Javel for 20 litres of water, and explained carefully that the bleach is not poisonous when one uses as little as one drop per litre. To prove this, the Motivators were the first to drink the treated water. Then the Care Group members were no longer afraid, and all tasted the chlorinated water.

From there, the Care Groups and Motivators went on to organise village meetings to teach everybody about cholera, and what to do to prevent or to treat it. At one place the local traditional healer headed the meeting. It was interesting to see that it was him who motivated the people to adopt the method. We were happy that the whole community would now be able to have safe water.

But there were some problems. Not even all the Care Group members were using the method at home, even if they would have liked to. One reason was a belief, coming from the elderly people at home, that Javel bleaches your intestine. The grannies even thought the young mothers wanted to get rid of them so that they and their husbands could stay alone at home. They said, 'That is why they put Javel in the water – to get rid of the old people.'

The Song of Cholera

On 17th December
Mr. Masilane came
He taught us about cholera.

When we see a person vomit,
When we see a person having
diarrhoea,
This is cholera.

Cholera finishes the body's strength,
The body's water and salts.

We shall prevent it!
Build a toilet and pass stools there
Build it far from the springs.
Wash your hands when you come
from there.
Wash your hands before touching
food.

We will protect ourselves!
By washing our hands.
By digging a rubbish pit
To throw the refuse there.

We will protect ourselves!
By boiling the drinking water
Or by adding a small teaspoonful
of Javel or Jik.
To 25 litres of drinking water.

We will protect ourselves!
By washing the vegetables
In clean water.
By washing each fruit
Before eating it.

Risimu ra cholera

Siku leriya ti 17th n'weti leyi ya
December
Ku fikili tatana Masilane
kambe hina hi dyondzisiwile.

Loko hi vona munhu a sungula
a hlanta,
Loko hi vona munhu a sungula
ku chuluka,
Hi yona cholera.

Cholera yi n'wi heta matimba,
mati na mimunyu e mirini.

Hi ta yi sivela!
Aka xiyindlana xa ku hambukela
kona.
Xi akiwa kule na xihlovo.
Hlamba mavoko u huma kona.
Hlamba mavoko u nga si khoma
swakudya.

Hi ta tisivela
hi ku hlamba mavoko.
Ku cela godi ro chela thyaka.

Hi ta tisivela
hi ku virisa mati yo nwa,
Kumbe ku chela xilepulana xa
Javel kumbe Jik
e matini yo nwa ya 25 liter.

Hi ta tisivela
hi ku hlantswa miroho
hi mati yo tenga.
Hlantswa mihandzu
u nga si yi dya.

Cholera is terrifying us.	Cholera ya chavisa va ka hina.
It is terrifying.	Ya ku chavisa
We will protect ourselves!	*Hi ta tisivela.*
We will protect ourselves!	*Hi ta tisivela*
When a person has diarrhoea and vomits,	Loko munhu yi n'wi komile wa chuluka a hlanta
Take her to the hospital quickly.	A yisiwe e xibedleni i xihatla.
Give her *tiribi* * all the time.	Nwisa tiribi minkarhi hinkwayo.
We will protect ourselves!	*Hi ta tisivela*
It is better to prevent.	Swa antswa ku sivela.
We thank you, our Motivators.	Ha nkhensa varhangeri!

* THE CARE GROUPS' NAME FOR ORAL REHYDRATION FLUID

4. The Care Groups increase and multiply: 'We forgot to do family planning'

It was not possible to stop new groups forming, because people were pushing. I think they saw how successful it was. They saw people treating themselves and improving their homes, while they themselves still had their problems of trachoma, diarrhoea and other preventable diseases. They felt they could do the same if they had Care Groups. As I always say, 'The Care Group Movement is a mother that did not do family planning'. That is why so many children were born without preparation. There were too many, and we couldn't handle them. And there were no plans to cope with the growth of the project. We just thought of the problems we could see. We did not think of the future, and we did not know that the groups would have demands – more and more.

Chapter 3

The Care Groups come of age

Vuxaka bya tin'hwari i ku handza swin'we

Partridges become friends by scratching the ground together

Distribution of Care Groups in former Gazankulu in 1996.
(Drawn by U. Knecht, based on a map in 'A Development Framework for Gazankulu';
Institute for Development Studies, Rand Afrikaans University, 1983)

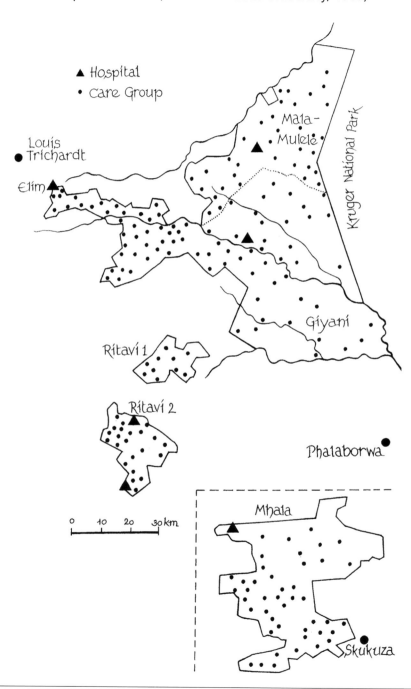

Chapter 3

The Care Groups come of age

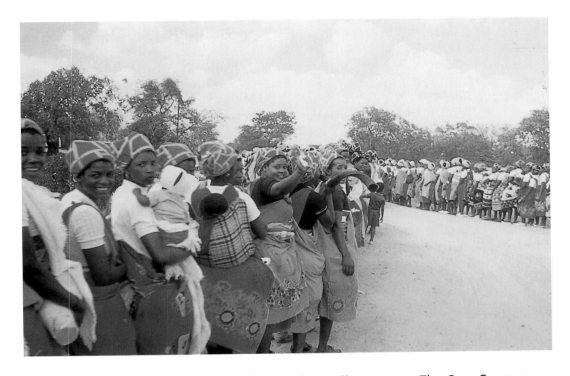

Waiting for the Eye Doctor to arrive for her farewell ceremony. The Care Groups organised the function on their own. They are proud that they can take many things into their own hands. (Photo: L. Karlsson)

Eight years after the first Care Groups were founded, Erika Sutter retired and left Elim. In 1983 a new doctor, Carel IJsselmuiden, who is a Community Health specialist, joined the team for three years. A Project Co-ordinator was also appointed. A Community Health Office was opened in Elim in the mid-1980s, and the Care Groups had their own office there.

During the first eight years, the groups gained valuable experience of organising and working together, and they had already extended their work beyond trachoma control to include a wide variety of projects to promote general health and development. With the new team leadership, more emphasis was laid on the empowerment of Motivators and groups. Leadership, planning and evaluation were stressed. The groups embarked on more new activities, including income-generating schemes which sometimes threatened to displace health as a major concern.

The groups and the Motivators began to gain the confidence to act on their own, and the time was ripe to set up structures which would make the Care Groups more independent of the hospitals, and give more responsibility to the groups and their elected committees. Each Health Ward now has its Care Group council composed of delegates from the groups. The council in turn chooses a management committee, called the 'Top Executive', which takes care of the area's Care Groups. This change had already been suggested in the early 1980s, but the groups were not yet ready for it. Even at the end of the first eight years, the development was not entirely smooth.

Looking into the future, there are discussions going on about the Care Group movement becoming a non-government organisation (NGO), separate from the Government's health services. A Care Group Training Centre was opened at the end of 1999.

Discussing the next step is the responsibility of the Care Groups Transition Committee, which has members from the communities, chosen by the project management and the Top Executives. However, as Selina Maphorogo writes, 'Even if the Project does eventually become completely independent of the Health Department as a non-governmental organisation, the groups will continue to involve the health services and give them a space.'

1. A new phase in the life of the Care Groups

When the Eye Doctor left it was a challenge. We wanted to show that we could keep the Care Groups going alone. When I told the groups she was leaving, the members were very disturbed. They asked, 'What will happen without her?' I asked them, 'How often have you seen her?' They answered, 'Oh, once or twice.' I said, 'You see. We pick all she has in her head and put it into our heads. And when she flies home to Switzerland, she will be quite light.' So they were happy.

The Care Group Motivators become more independent

At the beginning, I used to wait for the Eye Doctor to tell me what I should do. The doctor who took over later just kept quiet and said nothing when we were waiting for him to give orders. He wanted us to do things by ourselves. We had to be very clear ourselves about why we wanted to do a thing, because he was always questioning 'Why?' One day he wanted something from us that we did not agree with, and we asked, 'Why?' He was so surprised!

When we had workshops we learned to ask 'Why?' about things people wanted us to do, or things we did not understand. This taught me to stand up and say 'No' when somebody asks me to do something in the community that I know is not good. When I am really convinced, I can even say 'No' when I am asked to do something by someone in a higher position, until the reasons for doing it have been explained to me. I now have confidence in myself, and I feel strong because I do not work alone, but I work with other people. The women in the Care Groups and we, the Motivators, are getting stronger every day and we have learned how to solve our problems. We have learned to stand up when things are tough.

When we had workshops we learned to ask 'WHY'? (Photo: E. Sutter)

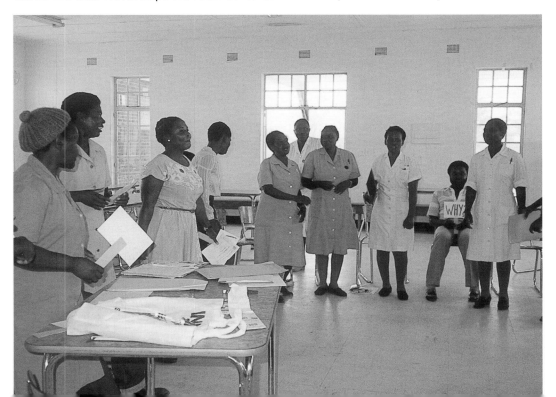

2. A new structure: the Care Groups form their own association

In the 1980s, senior people working with the Care Groups thought it would be a good thing for Care Group members to have their own organisation where they could be more independent of the hospital. The members and the Motivators were told to take steps to introduce a Care Group Association, but none of them were really clear about what was to be done. When the Motivators were trying to start the Care Group Councils and their Top Executives, the members thought that the Motivators were dumping the groups.

At that time, the groups were used to being dependent on the hospital. It really was a problem. The members feared that the Motivators would not be coming to the community any more – they thought that they were going back to work in the hospital. This caused a little bit of confusion, and many people thought they would no longer want to belong to this movement. They thought the Care Group would carry the whole load, and the community would blame them for not doing anything. We needed some tough discussions to make people understand what it was all about. The problem was that the idea did not come from the groups themselves, but from the Project Management.

The structure that was finally introduced was like this. In each Health Ward, every Care Group sends two members to the Care Group Council. The senior Motivators are there as advisors. The Councils then choose 7 people to become members of a management committee, called the 'Top Executive'. Each member is responsible for 4–6 groups in her area.

When I got back from training in England, I did not go to visit the groups so much, but spent a lot of time with the members of the Top Executive, training them for their job. I was pushing the point that it was not for them alone to take decisions, but that they should always work together with the groups.

The Care Group members and Top Executive members are working together more and more. The members are very proud of being more independent and are taking many things into their own hands. The Top Executive is very active. They have their own bank account, and have managed to raise some funds from selling peanuts and soups. They are encouraging bulk buying, and they manage a peanut bulk buying scheme (see page 139) completely on their own. They are in charge of the loans for Care Groups who need funds to complete projects.

A new structure for the Care Groups. (Drawing: Victoria Francis)

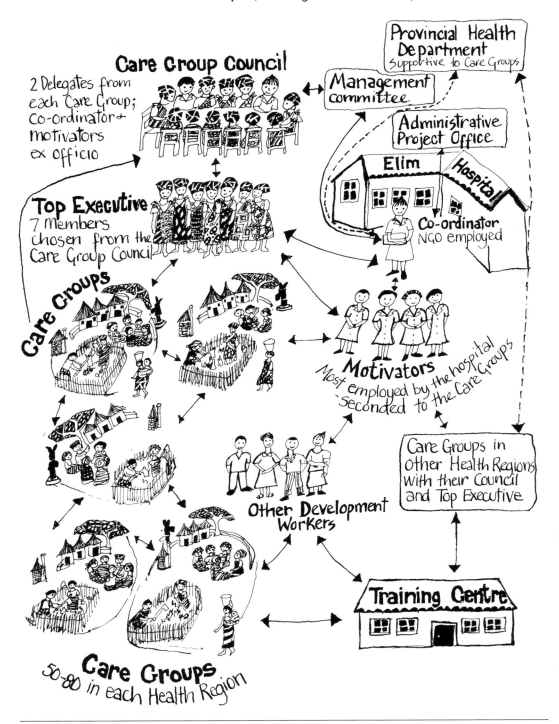

Provincial Health Department
Supportive to Care Groups

Care Group Council
2 Delegates from each Care Group; Co-ordinator + motivators ex officio

Management committee

Administrative Project Office

Elim Hospital

Top Executive
7 Members chosen from the Care Group Council

Co-ordinator
NGO employed

Care Groups

Motivators
Most employed by the hospital — seconded to the Care Groups

Other Development Workers

Care Groups in Other Health Regions with their Council and Top Executive

Training Centre

Care Groups
50-80 in each Health Region

In the beginning I did not like the name 'Top Executive', but now I like it, because we see them as being on top of the Motivators, and I respect them as being my superiors who can tell me what they want me to do. I am very happy that the first step to what we were looking forward to long ago has been made, and that the members organise things for themselves. For example recently the Care Group members organised a meeting to which they invited the Top Executive members of the six Health Wards. They catered for the meeting themselves, and did not ask the Project to do the catering. They are also organising a refresher course for Care Group members, and are only involving us for advice.

3. A new role for the Motivators

Encouraging the group's own decisions: 'We know what we want'

Nowadays, we find that many Care Groups have a very good understanding and that they can help the community to be aware of their problems. When we take enough time to sit down with the group and discuss community problems with the members, we find that they come up with very good solutions. Really, the Care Group members have grown up! That is why I think it is right that the Care Group members should chose whether they still want to go for Care Groups or do something else. These days they know exactly what they want. They cannot be pushed from place to place any more.

It can happen that some groups stop meeting for a time. There are many reasons for this. For example, one group stopped Care Group work some years ago, because they had heard about a new co-operative which was starting at the Tribal Office. They were able to say straight away that they were no longer coming to the Care Group, because they were busy with that other project. This is much better than when we always went to the Care Groups with our own decisions, and they just said, 'Yes, yes, yes', and forced themselves to do a thing which would not last.

There is another group where the team is very strong. When they decide to stop meeting for a while, they stop. Even if you go there and want to have a meeting, they will not come. That is the way they want to function. But when they decide they want to meet again, or to do something together, they do come. When they need to fetch wood from far away, they go together, in a team, to hire a car together to carry the wood.

Some people may think that these Care Groups are not functioning well. This is not true – they do function. If they think they have nothing to discuss, why should they meet? It is no use pushing people. Often, even while the groups are not meeting, they still stick together and people still ask them for advice.

I respect the people and what they say – so if they don't want to meet when I go to their village I go round the community and do house visiting instead. And when I see something that it would be good for the group to know, I will come up with it when we meet next time. Maybe some Motivators might think if there is no Care Group meeting, 'Why should I still go there?' But people must know that the Motivators are there. We should keep their friendship and trust – and when they want to have meetings again, then we will go to meet with them. We are not wasting time, even though it may sometimes look like that to our superiors, who don't understand what is happening in the community. The hospital expects us to write formal reports about meetings with the groups. We do write informal reports about what we have actually done – which may be house visiting or another activity, not a group meeting – but that is not what they want to hear about.

Care Groups are passing on their experience to other organisations

Many people are realising that the style the Care Groups are working in is appropriate, and other organisations are now copying what the Care Groups are doing. They are training groups of people to start small projects, and those Care Group members who joined these groups can help them, as they already have a lot of experience. Elderly Care Group members are also very active in an organisation helping the aged, which is present in several communities. Care Group members are training the others. For example, one elderly lady has been taught how to plant fruit trees, and now she has a nursery where she trains other elderly people. Even the Government's Community Development Department and the Department of Agriculture are adopting the method of group action. These are great steps the Care Groups have achieved.

Do the groups still need Motivators ?

Now that the Care Groups are organising more and more on their own, some people are asking whether we Motivators are still needed. They even suggest that we should go back to work in the hospital and leave the groups struggling on their own, and that this would be the best way for the women to learn!

We have had some groups who did not know what to do when the Motivators were not there. But many others do different things when the Motivator is not there, for example looking after the sick and old in their community. One group went on their own initiative to examine the school children for trachoma, and at another time they went to examine them for scabies and advised them what to do. After an accident happened with a child eating the fruits of a poisonous tree people like to plant for shade, one group went round to inform all the families about the dangers of that tree, and then the tree was destroyed.

If people know what they want, they can do things themselves. But even groups that can work independently, taking their own decisions, can still benefit from Motivators who will come in if needed. Motivators can help with their knowledge, and guide the Care Group in planning in order to achieve its aims. Therefore Motivators are still needed.

4. Projects for income or projects for better health?

Around the time of the 10th anniversary of the Care Group Project people got more interested in job-creating projects than in health. Because many of them were poor, they tried to solve their problem of poverty in this way. They started things like small brickyards or sewing groups. Some Care Groups were dropping health completely. But how can people work if they are not healthy? The two should go together. Even if they are working in a brickyard, the women should still manage to have a small garden where they can grow green vegetables. With some people, when they get money, what happens? Instead of buying healthy food, they go for the food which is easy. They buy bread and cool drinks, which is not healthy. They will not think of yellow fruit – they have no time to think of all these things, they are busy thinking about money. Some of the groups stopped sharing with their community when they had their job-creating projects. Members of the Top Executive were very much aware of the problem. During a refresher course they talked about it:

'When we have projects like brick-making they can be good for the community. But with some brick-making projects the community is not helped by getting cheaper bricks. People from outside buy the bricks, and the group alone earns the money. Some groups are only busy with sewing and selling, and they are not interested in anything that is happening in the community. People in the community say, "Those people who have a lot of money started the Care Groups. So let those who have money go for Care Groups. We did not get anything." This destroys the team spirit. They are selfish when they do not let other people in, poor people who need a job.

'Those groups who keep the projects for themselves have even stopped going to Care Group meetings. They don't think about their health, their children or their neighbours any more. They no longer look at things the same way. They only think of the project and making money. They only attend the meetings where there is a plan for funds. If it is a meeting about health, they don't attend. People begin to have wrong expectations of the Care Groups. They think it is to get a job. But we who are seeing the values of the Care Groups, we really feel we are going to continue.'

Health is still a concern – and the groups are taking more responsibility

Today most Care Groups have learned to have income-generating projects without neglecting health. While the Care Groups are involved in all these little projects, they continue to work closely together with the health services.

The women have taken many health issues into their own hands. They come up with demands and want to know more. They have seen that progress has happened through prevention; they are willing to promote health and watch to see whether the health points are functioning well. Health education in the community will not stop. This is why the Care Groups go on and on.

5. 'Still with Care Groups after more than 25 years': Voices of Care Group members

We wanted to know what Care Group members themselves think about the Movement and why they are still with the Care Groups after more than 25 years. At refresher courses we asked members of the Top Executive and other Care Group members to divide into small groups, and the groups were asked to draw a picture of the Project.

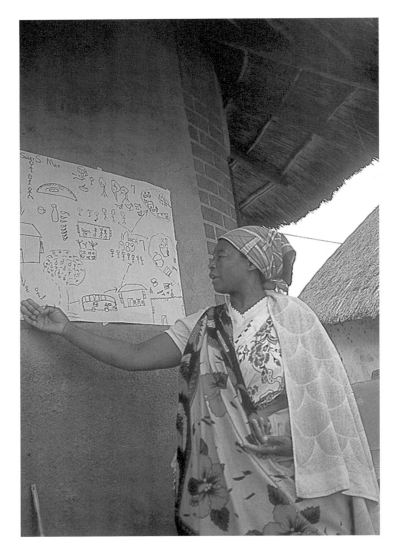

A member explains her group's picture. (Photo: E. Sutter)

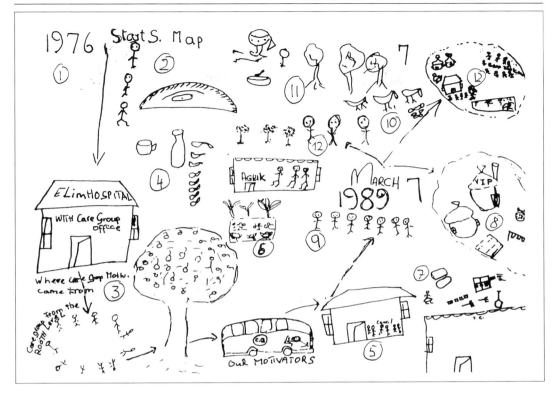

Picture of the Care Group Project drawn by a group of members.

Explanation:

1 Care Groups started in 1976 with Selina Maphorogo, Mr Radebe and Dr Sutter
2 We started with eyes
3 You came down from the hospital, sitting with us under the big tree
4 We learnt many things, like how to make Oral Rehydration Fluid
5 Later the Care Group met in the Tribal Office
6 We learned vegetable gardening
7 We learned to make Wonder Boxes
8 We built VIP toilets
9 In March 1989 the seven "Top Executive" members were elected
10 We also learnt how to make chicken runs
11 We planted Leucaena trees
12 The Top Executive looks after all the Care Groups in our area

Xivongo Shandlani	@ Bag RB Saekmebaaxs liniki	Siku			1.8.83	19.83	1.10.83	1.11.83			Machupa ya mishi
		Vito	sex	age	+	+	+	+	+	+	
		John.	M	7½	+	O	O	O			
		Dayina	♀	45	0	O	O	O			Xivodwana X (toilet)
		Anna.	♀	20	0	O	O	O			Xithopa x (garden)
		Rose	♀	10	0	O	O	O			Xikalu xa Vaaa ✓ (UF clinic)
		Mukelani.	M	1	+	+	+	+			gedji to chela
		Xaniseka.	M	2	+	+	O	O			typhaka X (refuse pit) ✓
		Violet	♀	20	0	O	O	O			Swithawulana (face cloths)

Page from a member's notebook.

'Before, we were too shy to join anything we were not used to. Now we attend literacy classes.' 'We also learned to keep records of "our" families whom we visited' (*Care Group Members*). (Photo: I. Bourcart)

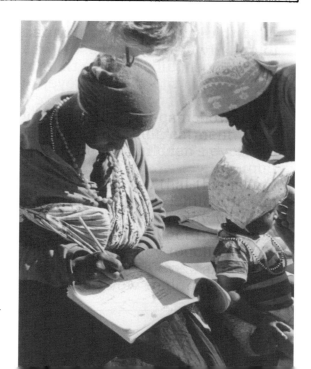

New knowledge and new self-confidence

When we started we were scared to go to the clinic; now we do go. Before, we were too shy to join anything we were not used to. Now we attend literacy classes. We also learned to preserve different types of food and to make spices. Even our husbands were very impressed with the new recipes and wanted to know where we learned it. Now they say, "Never stop going to the Care Group, because they are teaching you good things". Before, our husbands did not come home from town for six months. Now they come every month. This is very important for us.

All this has happened because people from the hospital came down to us, sitting with us under the big tree. They came down, not remaining high up in the hospital.

Health, community development and women's self-reliance

Care Groups are still alive because we have seen that when we are working in a group we get ideas from each other and find solutions towards solving our problems, because women have similar worries, such as problems caused by husbands or children. We can only be successful by working together, meeting together. During our meetings we have long discussions and try to solve our problems. And when the problem is too big, we discuss it with members of other community committees. We see changes in the community because people have learned how to handle many of their problems.

We are also starting to change our relationship with the men. Traditionally, when a woman speaks in a meeting, men do not listen, and they object. But this is the New South Africa. So things must change. They must get used to it that women have good ideas and should talk. It is not like before. Men should start listening to women and accept it when they have a good point. Some men see the good points of Care Groups. Observant men can see the changes in their homes. Now we talk freely with our husbands – before, we were afraid to talk. Those who have been beaten are no longer beaten. We also take good care of our hair and clothes, just like those women in the big cities. This has helped to persuade many of our

Chapter 4

The Care Groups at work

1. What makes a Care Group function well?

'What is important is the behaviour of the leader'

I have seen that for any project, what is important is the behaviour of the leader, whether the leader is from the community or from outside. If a person is too powerful, once this person says something, the others all follow. People need a steady person who can listen and will find out together with the people what can be done to solve a problem. Sometimes what we think about a leader in the community may be wrong. We might say, 'Oh, this chairlady is a very good person. She is so active'. And then we find that she made all the decisions on her own, not involving the group.

It is difficult to find a solution to the problem of unsuitable leaders in the Care Groups. The issue was discussed in a Care Group members' refresher course, and the members came to the conclusion that it would be best if chairladies were to be changed every two years. This would give more people a chance to learn to be a leader. Also, with rotating leadership a too-powerful chairlady could be replaced without offending her. But in practice it has not worked. The old chairlady feels that it would not be nice for her to become an ordinary member again, and the members who trust her may feel that if she is not the one leading, it will not be nice any more. Rotating leadership worked only in one place, where people understood. There, the old chairlady is still giving advice to the new one.

An over-active chairlady makes it hard for the members to develop initiative

The chairlady of one Care Group was a very active person and was doing quite a lot of things in her community. She had some sewing groups, she was the leader of the Gazankulu Government's Women's Association and of various women's clubs. Everything that was on, she was in it. So when the Care Group started at her place, it was natural that she had to be the chairlady. In the Care Group she did all the planning. The group did not do any planning. Each time when the Motivators went there for training the Care Group on their meeting day, we were told that this was not the day for Care Groups, it was the day for cooking, or another time it was for sewing. There were too many things on the go. That is why that group was not functioning well. They couldn't do one thing at a time and only after this was finished, do something else. As the chairlady was an important person in the community, nobody could say they did not want her to be the chairlady. She was educated and was thinking that the Care Group members, who were less educated, could not do things on their own. For one refresher course, it was made clear that each group should send two ordinary members, not people from the committee. But this chairlady came too, saying, 'I must see what my children are doing'.

After that chairlady moved to another area it took a long time for the members to decide on action without her. Later the group was doing well, after they had learned the hard way to become independent. They have some job creation projects and they built a VIP toilet at the market place where the taxis park. They allocated themselves to a rota for cleaning the toilet every day. They talked to the taxi committee about paying the people who were cleaning around the toilet. Because of the market and the taxi rank which are there, there is a lot of rubbish lying around. The Care Group also did street cleaning.

It can also happen that there is a group of persons directing everything. In one of the Care Groups some members were school teachers. The chairlady was a teacher, and those organising the group were also teachers. In the beginning I liked going to that group so much. When I arrived I found that they were so organised, because the teachers who were leading knew how to run meetings. The only thing I had to do was to explain about the disease and how they should go about treating it. The teachers organised and planned and told the illiterate members, 'You go there, and you go to that other area and do the house visits'.

It was so easy for us! But now when I think of it I know it was not correct, because those who were not so well educated did not have a chance to open their mouths. They were not involved in the planning. The teachers did not do the work in the families, but they were praised for the good work the group did. When the time came that the teachers left, the other members of the group felt lost, because they had never been involved in discussions and did not know how to plan.

Ordinary Care Group members can accomplish a lot

An ordinary Care Group member can be very effective and can improve the work of the group. It is often a person who is already involved in a lot of things. Some of them are very clear about what they want to do and what they don't want. It makes me feel happy to work with these people.

In the group I have described above, there was just one member who remained active after the teachers had left. She kept on going house visiting and could help the other families when they had problems. She motivated the group to check whether the mothers took their children to the child health clinic and if they had the 'Road-to-Health' chart, and to find out if the children were immunised against measles. It worked very well. When there were some problems, she could help the members by sitting down with the clinic nurse to solve them.

In another group, there was a member who used to go visiting people on the poorer side of her community, and people liked her and trusted her. She learned a lot about what was happening from going from house to house, because she was observing well. She was the one who was going to the chief for the people. When the hospital decided there should be a visiting point for the mobile clinic in her place, she looked after it. At that time there was no water there, but she managed alone to keep this place going. She worked a long time without being paid for her work and never complained. Because of all these things she did, she was chosen to be trained as a Community Health Worker.

2. Case histories: two groups out of many ...

Like all organisations, Care Groups have their ups and downs. A group can be very busy and united sometimes, and then become very quiet when the members are tired of what they are doing – but if they have a special issue which is urgent for them and they want to do it, they can overcome difficulties. Then they push to do it. This section tells the stories of two of the many groups.

The energetic Care Group in X

The Care Group in X is an example of a group which has been functioning well from the time it started (1976) until today. It is an active group. Things they see that they should do, they do. At the time when we started, they did not have a big problem with trachoma. But they had problems with typhoid. There was a river, and they had enough water to wash themselves, but they did not have clean water to drink. They could not boil the water, because they did not have enough wood. So they preferred to use Javel fluid to disinfect the water. In all the houses they visited the Care Group members advised people to use it, and explained that there was no danger if it was used correctly.

When we were discussing their needs, it came out that they wanted to help sick people and the aged. The group allocated jobs to its members; someone was going for food, some were collecting water, some went to the homes of the aged or sick people to clean their things or washed the blankets. There was one old man who died of typhoid, and the whole family was admitted to hospital. When they came back from the hospital, Care Group members took care of that family, helping them to be clean, and advising them about clean drinking water.

There was one old lady who at the time of forced removals had refused to move with her family to another village, and she remained alone in X. One day her house collapsed. The Care Group members looked for grass for roofing, and some made bricks, and they built her a little house. They were also advising everyone to build toilets. The ground slopes so much in that place that they could not make the normal toilets, but they found a way of solving that problem. At that time we were not yet teaching people how to build toilets.

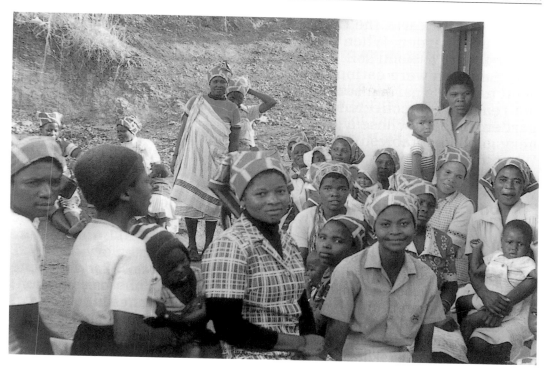

A Care Group in front of the Health Point they prepared for their community. (Photo: M. Kearney)

The community of X was very isolated. There was no public transport passing there and there was no clinic. When people were sick, they had to hire a car to reach the hospital or the next clinic. Also, when it was raining, the road was too slippery and cars could not pass. So the group decided they would make a visiting point for the mobile clinic from the hospital. They asked the shopkeeper for a storeroom, and then they made some windows and white-washed the walls. One Care Group member brought a bed, and another one a table, and others came with some chairs. After the Care Group members had finished painting, and the mobile clinic started to come, an important man in the community was so happy that he slaughtered a goat for the Care Group members. There was a big feast, and they invited everybody. This is something that gives courage, when the community members see the work of the Care Group. Many years later a new visiting point was built, and there the Care Group members made a good VIP toilet. That is how the Care Group in X improved life for their community.

again. They planted peanuts, but unfortunately there were lots of termites and nothing was growing. So they said, 'We told you! There is a lot of witchcraft!' And next year, again nothing was done in the garden. It went on and on like that.

Then at last they decided to get started. The Agricultural Extension Officer (AEO) was prepared to teach them. Then the rain came and people started ploughing, but the group did not have any money on hand. When the chairlady saw a man ploughing with a tractor in the neighbourhood, at a cheap price, she tried to call a meeting, but she could not find anybody that day. She thought, 'That man with the cheap tractor will now go somewhere else and it will be difficult to get him back'. So she asked him to plough the garden for the Care Group, and said that the group would pay him later. So he ploughed. And when she told the group that the garden had been ploughed, and what had to be paid, some of them said, 'We are not paying that money. Who told you to hire that tractor?'

From that time on the group was divided and was fighting all the time. The AEOs asked us to help them. They did not know what to do and did not manage to bring the people together. The women were so quarrelsome that the AEOs were afraid that they would start to fight physically. I was really scared that day we went there. I did not have anything in my mind as to what I could tell these people. I thought, 'I will hear from them while we are discussing'. We Motivators and the AEOs went together.

When we arrived there, those who were refusing to pay for the tractor were sitting next to each other, and the others were sitting on the other side. We let each side tell its story, and we were listening and not interfering. One group told us that when they were going to work in the garden, the others would also come and say that the garden belonged to all, and they could not be excluded from sowing seeds in it – but they were not going to pay for the tractor. So we asked, 'How do you want your garden to be when all the mealies around have germinated, and only you have nothing, but it is ploughed?' Then they started to quarrel. It was a big noise. I thought it was better to keep quiet for a while and let them quarrel as long as we were there, and see that they did not fight physically. I thought, if we were scared and left them when they quarrelled, it would never change. And if we told them to stop, they would just start again after we had left. When people are quarrelling, it is better just to stay there till they stop on their own.

When they were tired, I said, 'Let us look now and see if what we are doing is making us reach somewhere. What does the community think of us, when we are a Care Group and are making such a lot of noise, we are quarrelling and are pointing fingers at each other? Are we helping our community to recognise our good work?' Then it was so quiet!

So I asked them, 'Are you now prepared to talk to each other without shouting, so that I can hear what you are saying?' We tried to guide the discussion, so that they managed to say all they felt they should say. Then I asked, 'What do you think should be the end of it? Are we letting the garden become a grazing place, because when some want to plant, the others say no?'

They were quiet for a while. The AEO explained that it was still not too late to plant a crop. After a long discussion the question about the tractor was settled, and they all paid their share. Finally, I said, 'Well, I don't know whether you will get together, or how you are going to show the community which type of Care Group you are. As far as we are concerned, beyond listening to what you have been talking about, there is nothing we can do about it. It is your garden.' Now they started talking to each other about how they could get seeds, how will they go about it, when they were going to plant, and so on. Then I asked them, 'What are you going to do next time?' They made a good plan. They said that they would keep the money in one place, and elect a person to look for a tractor, but they must know who will go and what she will do.

The AEOs said to us, 'We are very thankful that everything is settled. We hope you will come again when we call you to help to solve problems. We were confused and did not know how to guide these discussions. We were afraid even to come to the garden.' And we said, 'It was a pleasure for us. We also will call on you, so that we can help each other.' We left it to the AEO to advise them about seeds and so on.

From then on, the group was all right. In the end, they also managed to build the reservoir. They even said, 'We really apologise for what we did when we were eating the money before. If we had taken the advice and acted on it, we would have a lot of money now. Now we have to pop out money. It is such a lot of money. But we are going to try and do it.' They worked very hard, and when they were short of money again, they went together to earn some, and put it in a common fund. When the reservoir was half finished, they asked for advice about how to finish it. I suggested that they should write letters to local people, asking for funds, and they did that. Finally, I helped them with some money I still had from some ladies in Switzerland who knew about Care Groups. I said, 'It is not my money, I did not work for it. This is other people's money. I will write and tell them how it is going to be used. And if you waste it, it is other people's money you are misusing!'

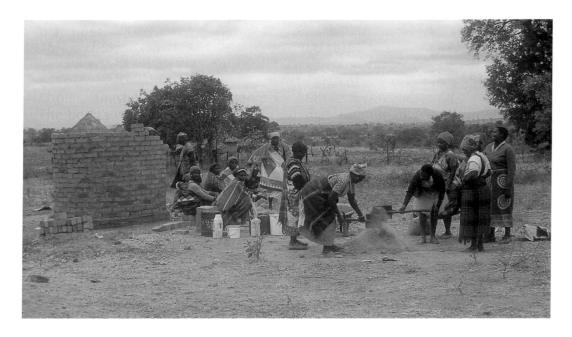

A Care Group building a water reservoir. (Photo: P. Kok)

At first, the group did not want to share their reservoir with the rest of the community, because they had paid for everything and done all the work. But what could be done about the rest of the village, which did not have any water? Finally, the group decided to build another reservoir, nearer to the houses. They will not build it on their own this time. The whole community will be involved in paying for the tank and piping. The solar pump of the communal garden, which was already there, could be used for both reservoirs. The Care Group will share the water with the community. So they have learned to share with the community, and not only improve things for themselves!

3. Care Groups carrying out projects

Projects should come from the Care Groups themselves

In the beginning we did not know ourselves how to go about carrying out projects, but we have learned from the mistakes we have seen, and from those we have made ourselves. For example if we tell a Care Group to start a project which came from the Motivator's mind, and the members are assured that they will earn money, people will expect everything from the Motivators. People will think it is the Motivators' project, not their project. It is not good when organisers rush into projects. Projects should be things that come from the Care Groups themselves. It is best if the people think about what they want and work on a plan of how it should function. I have seen many projects – some good ones, and some that failed. Here, I describe some of them, and others are to be found in other chapters of the book.

One example of a project that did not reach its target-group was a child nutrition project organised by some doctors, together with the chiefs, the teachers and the nurses at the clinic. The people who really needed the weaning food (a porridge made with maize flour and ground peanuts) were not involved. They were not with it from the start, and they had no say. No one wanted to grind the peanuts and the beans. The Care Group mothers did not see any reason why they should keep organising, because those who were in the committee, the chiefs and the teachers, were those who had everything they needed. They were not the people who needed the scheme. And the people who really needed the porridge thought it was not for them. They thought the project was for the teachers, because they organised it. And the teachers thought that the poor families who needed the porridge were very low people. In this way it couldn't work. Yet the people in that community were really in need of the project. There was a lot of malnutrition.

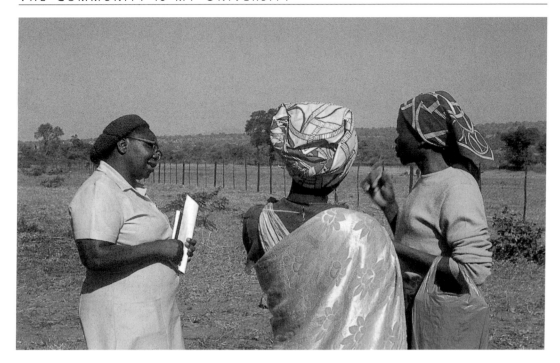

'It is best if people themselves think about what they want with a project and work on a plan of how it would function.' Here, a communal garden is being discussed. (Photo: E. Sutter)

One can also make mistakes by doing a good project with the wrong group. There was one place where the Care Group had already started a small project, sewing wonder boxes. But instead of assisting this group, which had tried to do something by themselves, we started with wonder boxes in another community and supported the new group. The group which had worked hard to start on the sewing and had already put some money into the project was very unhappy about it.

We have to observe better. We have to do things at the correct time and at the correct place, so that the right people are supported with funds.

Projects should give people a chance to learn

At one time, under the old Government, people from a Government Department had some special funds for development, and they went into a community telling people that they would give them money to start a sewing project which could provide them with some income. A group of women was interested in taking part in this project. The project organisers bought them two sewing machines and a knitting machine, and wool and material. The women were not given funds to buy things for themselves. They had only to make a list of all they needed, and then the Government would buy the material and bring it to them. All the money was kept by the Government office, and the women were not allowed to go and choose the things they wanted themselves. They were even not told how much money was left for their project.

The women made some garments and sold them. All the money went back to the office, and the women were paid according to the products they made. One day those in charge of that development fund said that the money was finished and they could no longer provide them with material. And the group stopped functioning.

If they had had somebody to discuss project management with them and teach them about bookkeeping, they could have kept the money they were earning together, and they would have known where their money was going. The money the group got after selling their products would have gone back to them to buy new material and keep on sewing. They could always have put enough money aside for the material they needed before paying out the money that was left as earnings. In this way they could have continued with their own project, because they would have been educated to budget and to organise themselves. They would not have had to depend on the Government office where they did not know what had been done with the money.

I do not know whether development officials who work like this are really developing the community. If things are done for the project, people never get a chance to learn by themselves and will always depend on Government officials or other development organisations. The project will never grow. Community development needs action by the people themselves.

A promising project spoilt by too much pressure to show results

One Care Group made their own little survey, visiting all the families
in their community to find out what was worrying people most.
They found that many mothers were working in a tea plantation.
They were absent from home all day and had to leave their young
children behind with the grandmothers, who were unable to feed
them properly or to take them to the Child Health Clinic, which
was a long distance away. The children got malnourished and were
not checked at the clinic.

The group decided to ask the hospital to send a mobile child health
clinic to their village. The child health clinic came. After some
time the Care Group members realised that this was not enough.
The children remained malnourished. Then they thought of
organising a crèche for these children. They collected money
amongst themselves, and they learned how to write letters to raise
funds. They went to the shopkeeper, the taxi owner, and other
better-off people in the community and asked for help. The chief
gave them a site for the building. The group made bricks with a
small brick-making machine. They worked very hard, and had
already arranged with the community who would come and build,
once the bricks were ready. The whole time, the community was
very much behind the project and people were looking forward to
having a crèche.

However, because the Care Group members were doing everything
on their own, progress was slow. Some people from the project
management got impatient and asked for funds for building the
crèche. Some donors promised funds, but they wanted to know
what the project would cost and how far it had got. They set time
limits and asked for progress reports.

The Care Group was pushed to finish the building. A building team
from outside was hired, and bricks bought. It was still too slow for
the donors, and the responsibility for running and organising the
project was taken away from the Care Group. This was damaging
for them and for the community. People were no longer interested,
and the building was vandalised before it was completed. The
group was discouraged. For many years there were troubles about
ownership of the project and about who should be responsible for
running it.

A success-story: 'My favourite project'

There is one project which really makes me happy. It is a centre for the aged. It is a very interesting story. One day a lady from England contacted me. She wanted to start something in our area. She did not tell me what type of work she did; she just wanted to listen first and know what is happening in the area. We sat down

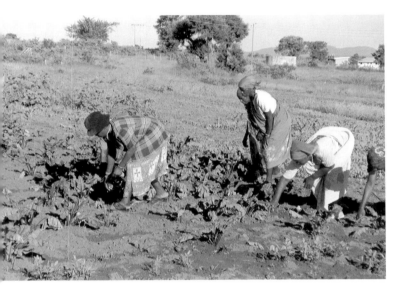

'My favourite project'. A group of elderly people planned and worked on their own garden, assisted by the local Care Group. Now they are producing vegetables like the sweet potatoes in the lower picture. (Photos: M. Morier-Genoud)

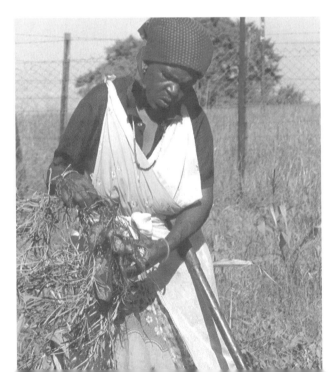

together and talked, and I explained what we were doing. And the last thing I mentioned was that for some years the members of a certain Care Group had kept on asking to start something with elderly people. But we ourselves had no skills to work with elderly people, so we would not know how to tell the Care Group members how to go about it. She said, 'Now I see that I am in the right place, because my job is to work with elderly people, running workshops.' That is how it came. She could have said, 'I want to go to the community to start a project for elderly people.' But because she listened first to what our needs were, I was able to explain to her some of the problems we come across with people who come from outside and want to do something in the community, and after a while they go and things remain flopping. That is why she then ran a workshop on participatory needs assessment together with the Motivators, the Care Group, and the members of the community, including the elderly people. She was not the one training the Care Group members – we were doing it. I think that is the best way of doing things. Even if the English lady goes away, the project will remain because the Motivators can continue with the project.

The elderly people came up with several ideas: for a garden project where they can plant the vegetables they like; health monitoring; care for the bedridden – and handicrafts, to show the young people how to do traditional crafts. Now people are really pushing for the project to be successful. They are struggling for themselves, and asking for assistance from us only when they think they need it. That is the proper way, it is going to be their project. It will not be the Motivators' project and it will not be my project. It is the community members who own it.

Now the old people have started to prepare their plot for a vegetable garden, where they want to plant those vegetables they like. When I went there to see how they are doing, they were busy putting up the fence. I stayed for some time, giving them a hand. They were working so hard, and it was so hot, that I was afraid someone would collapse. So I had to say, 'I am so tired, I need to have a rest', only to force them to make a break. Sometimes, when I ask them if I should do a certain task for them, they refuse and say, 'No, we will do it.' Then I have to sit back and let them do it.

They have managed to organise all the activities for themselves. Everything is in their hands. They have a centre where they can meet, and the old people are instructing the young ones in the old crafts, which are in danger of getting lost, and showing them the traditional dances. So old and young have fun together.

Different types of community workers are involved, all working together. The Motivators plan with the project members step by step, and train them in bookkeeping and to look after the money. They teach them how to care for sick, frail elderly people, about good nutrition and a good way of cooking. The Agricultural Extension Officers demarcated the land and advised the elderly people about good methods of planting crops according to the season. The Health Inspectors have shown them good places for building the toilets, where to build a *rondavel* to work and rest in, and a water reservoir, to avoid health hazards. The nurse at the Health Centre examines all members of the group, gives advice about diet, and treatment to those needing it, for example those with a sore back, knees or ankles, and those with high blood pressure or diabetes. The Social Worker helps those who need help with the pension fund, or have other social problems. When different sections plan together like they are doing in this project, they can solve the problems together, and there will be no misunderstandings.

4. Project financing

Funds from outside: empowerment or dependency?

The Drought Relief programme from the Government, which was a job-creating programme, made a communal garden with one of the Care Groups. People were hired to fence the garden and they were paid for it. When the plot was ready, the Agricultural Extension Officer did a lot of things the Care Group would normally have done, like hiring a tractor to plough, or buying seeds. The Care Group members could not plan and organise or come up with their own ideas. The Care Group in the neighbouring village also wanted a garden organised by the Government. They thought it would be easier and they would not have to pay. To help them to decide, I told them a little story:

'Imagine that you are at the shop, and somebody comes – somebody you don't know. He wants to buy bread, but his money is too little. He looks hungry. He wants to buy some bread, but he cannot even buy a quarter, because he is still 10 cents short. Then another person comes. He is hungry and goes around asking for food. You go out of the shop and there he is, asking you to give him a piece of bread, or some money. Which one would you help?'

They said, 'Oh, we think we would help the first one, the one who only asked for the 10 cents he was short of to buy the bread'.

I asked, 'Why?' Then there was a long discussion about doing all you can do yourself first, before you ask for help to finish the job you can't manage any more. Then the women realised the connection with their garden, and somebody asked, 'What will we do if the boys cut the wire from the fence to make their little cars? Who is going to repair it?' Finally they said, 'No, we don't want the Government one. They should only help us if we need it. We want to pay ourselves. We want to control the garden ourselves. With a Government garden we will have to write a report how the fence was cut and have to wait, and it will take too long for them to come and do the repair. If the garden is ours we will take care of it and see that the children are not going to cut the fences'.

I think this group was clever, because they wanted to have their own garden and do things their own way.

Funding should be offered when people have started something on their own

I don't think it is good to give money to a Care Group as soon as they think of beginning a small project. For example, right now there is one of the communities where the people are very much in need of peanuts for their children's weaning porridge. The group is thinking that if they had some funds, they would like to have their own bulk-buying scheme for peanuts, because at the shop they are too expensive. They would buy the peanuts from the farmers and sell them to people at a price they can afford. But I want first to see the group beginning something, and when I see they are well organised, then I can give them a revolving loan, and when they can sell their peanuts they will manage to bring some of the money back. Even if they don't manage to bring the whole amount, it will be something, and they will go on running their project for ever. The money which comes back will go to another group, and the money which comes back from that other group will go to the next, and so on. In this way we can help many groups.

Learning to manage resources

Projects should be an educational process. Before the Care Groups started with co-operatives, they did not know what to do with money they collected. They did not know where the money would be safe. They used to elect somebody who would keep the money on her body – but still no one knew if it was safe. And when a group was not sure whether they could trust the person who was keeping the money, at every meeting people would tell her, 'Let us see our money', and they kept on counting it.

Part of the education needed in a project is to teach people how to put the money into the bank. Then donations can go from the account of the Care Group Project Head Office straight into the bank account of the group that has a project. People can learn about interest and see how the interest is added to their accounts. If they want to do more than was originally budgeted for, they can work out how much they need to leave in the account or what needs to be added.

What many call development is not development when there is no education. If development does not go with education, people remain dependent on others. People learn from each of the different activities of the project. One must help people to think more about what they are doing and assist them when it is necessary – but not do things for them. We should do things with them so that later they can do them for themselves.

One of the Care Groups once got funds for building a water tank for the communal garden. They needed 25 bags of cement to make the bricks. The project supervisor told the group that she would go and buy the cement for them and look for transport and deliver it to them. Would it not have been better if she had gone with the women to town to go and buy the cement with them? Then they would have known where and how to buy cement, how to compare the prices and how to organise the transport. Later, they could have gone by themselves. If people organise supplies of things like sand and cement themselves and make bricks by themselves they learn how to go about it. Then they will be independent of other people such as the project supervisor. How can they learn if we buy everything and do everything for them? If we do, we are not helping a community project to continue and be an ongoing thing.

The problem is that progress is slow when people do everything on their own. Then some of us, especially the doctors and the managers, find it is too slow and they get nervous and want to push. But even if a project takes long, the people will be happy at the end, because it is really their own thing.

How can donors best support sustainable projects?

Many of the Care Group activities have always depended on donations from outside. I am happy that with the help of donors we can get some vehicles and that we can help many groups with funds when they don't manage on their own to reach their aims. In the early years, we Motivators were not involved in fund raising or in the allocation of funds to the different small projects. This was done by the Eye Doctor. Now the Motivators and the Care Groups themselves know much more about caring for their money, banking, keeping accounts and the proper way of applying for funds. Care Groups running a small project are now allowed to look after the money they receive themselves, and they have learned about its proper use.

One of our main donor organisations is the *Christoffel Blindenmission*, which has supported the Project since its early stages. Without them we could not have run the Project. They have a good way of dealing with us. Their field officer visits the Care Groups regularly. He knows the people who are involved in the Project and has a clear picture of what we are doing and what our needs are, and why we are applying for funds. Recently the Swiss *Département Missionnaire* has adopted the Care Groups as a partner organisation. They have provided equipment and are helping with some staff salaries. What I like about both these organisations is that they allow for sufficient time to organise step by step, discussing each step with all the people who are involved. In this way everyone is with us at each stage, and we have a better chance that the Care Groups will also continue in the future. Both these main supporters demand regular reports from us. This helps to educate the people in the Project to give feedback, and to use the funds properly.

However, with some other donors and outside development organisations we can get problems. There are some organisations that make all the plans for projects they are sponsoring. They decide that the project should start at this time and end at that time, because they want to see what we have done with their money. That makes us, as Motivators, feel we must push ahead, instead of doing things correctly with the people, step by step, with a lot of discussion. When we see that the finishing time the sponsors have set for the project is nearly there, then we push, because we are afraid that if we don't manage to give a report in time we will lose the funds. This damages the groups, because it is no longer an educational process.

The money is the problem. When such donors visit us they spend only a very short time with the project. They have quick discussions with us, without allowing us enough time to think of all the problems people might have when they want to organise their project. And when the money is already here, we can no longer tell the donors that the time has been too short and that we cannot start yet!

Planning should not be done by the donors only. Those who are actually involved in carrying out a project should first do their planning of the project. The donors will be kept informed about progress. We should really go back to our donors and tell them to leave us enough time for planning. Or, if the money has already been given they should allow us to keep it on one side until the project is well prepared, even if it takes 6–7 months. The donors may think this is a long time, but it is better for a project when people are clear about what they want to do before they start with something.

Chapter 5

The Care Groups in their communities

Vanhu i vukosi

People are the wealth of a chief

People are a gold mine

Chapter 5

The Care Groups in their communities

1. 'Care Groups are part of their communities'

Whatever is happening in a community, it will affect the groups. Sometimes it is helping them to function well, and at other times it may create problems for them.

Working in co-operation with the village authorities

Chiefs are part of traditional culture, ruling people in the village. The people in the village used to take care of the chief's family, because it was important to the community that the chief should stay in the village, and not go away to work elsewhere. The Apartheid Government interfered with the system. Tribal Offices were built to create a meeting place. The chiefs were paid by the Government, and the Government controlled the money for schools, clinics and so on. When apartheid ended, the Tribal Offices went on working, but together with an elected local government. Each community has its own civic group; people who represent all the structures and work hand in hand with the chief. In places where there were no chiefs, like Elim, there are elected Community Authorities.

At the beginning, when we Motivators wanted to start a Care Group or a project in a community, we always contacted the chief and explained what we wanted to do. If there were some people from his community who had already invited us to work with them, we would say that we had been called. If we had seen a problem ourselves, we would talk to the chief and ask him what he thought about the problem and what to do about it. And when he agreed to do something, we would offer to help him to explain it to the people. When I visit a group, I still often call at the chief's place, just to keep him informed. It is always good to involve the chief when starting in a community, as people depend on his goodwill and his support.

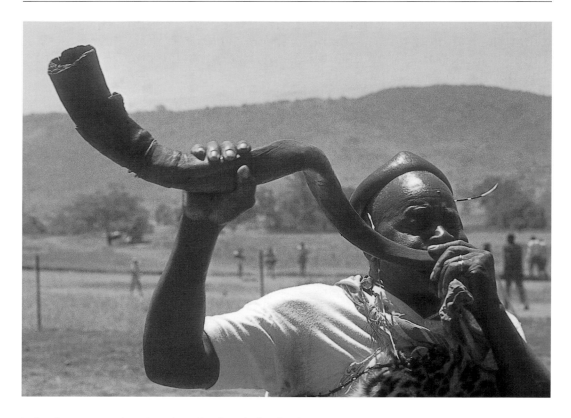

It is always good to involve the local chief when working in a community.
The picture shows a chief attending a Care Group function. (Photo: E. Sutter)

When the women come and sing and perform educational plays at
village gatherings, the chiefs can see that Care Groups are a good
thing. Now the Care Group members can also approach the chief
and ask for what they need. They know that the chief should be
notified about what they are doing, even when he is not an active
chief. In some places the women have gained in confidence and
are even able to fight for their group when the chiefs are
disturbing their work.

Working with the chiefs

When we started our work, the chief of one of the three pilot
communities understood very well when we explained about the
Project. He was there at the first meeting when we told the people

how to prevent trachoma. At that time we still used to tell people what they should do. It was not the people's own idea. But the chief now got this idea into his head, and he was giving courage to the people to do what they were supposed to do. So they became interested to go and tackle the disease.

But in a neighbouring place this didn't work. There, the women did not volunteer to join the Care Group, they were ordered by the chief to do the work. He allocated the duty of collecting eye ointment for the community to particular people. He was used to giving orders, and was thinking he was doing a good thing. Then some people complained to the chief that there was not enough ointment, and he started blaming those who had been told to collect it, although the real problem was that the hospital had no more supplies. That was not good.

Some chiefs are very helpful. There was one young chief who had a very good way of discussing things with people when the Motivators were absent. He supported them in whatever they wanted to do. When we organised a firewood plantation with the Care Group, we told the chief about it, and he was also happy. The members made the fence and planted the trees. It was a very interesting day, because everybody from the community was there. The chief was also there and was working with the people. That is why I say that this chief was very good, because I never saw another chief working with the people, digging and doing all these things. He was with the people and suffered with the people.

In places where the chief is very strong, and likes to tell the people what to do, the people can't do a thing without the chief. Such a chief may even be suspicious of the Care Groups. At one place the people in the Tribal Office invited us to go and see them, and they told us that they were unhappy that the Care Groups were taking power from the chiefs. They felt the Care Groups were the ones organising everything in the community. We discovered that the chiefs were afraid that the Care Groups could have more power in the community than they, the chiefs! This showed that Care Group members were working very hard and were doing something which everyone could recognise.

One Care Group thought of making a communal garden in order to produce some food to improve the health of their community. The garden was fenced and everything was all right. But while they were waiting for the rains to come, the chief thought of ploughing the garden for himself. The Care Group members decided to stand together to solve the problem. At first they wanted us to come and solve the problem with the chief. But we Motivators told them clearly that a person from outside does not belong to the community – they must be the ones to sort out the issue. There were lots of discussions to find out the right way to talk to the chief, and the members organised themselves and planned exactly who would say what. In this way they managed to win him to their side. He afterwards even helped them to finish the fencing of the plot and to get water. From then the women realised that, as a group, they were strong. This is women's empowerment.

Using all the community's resources: traditional healers

Health workers of all levels who are trained in the European way may think that they are the only ones who know how to treat patients, and they look down on the traditional healers who are called *sangoma*. Yet there are many things the *sangoma* know, and we should respect them. We do not think the same way as they do. I have many friends who are *sangoma*, and I tell them that my grandfather was one, too. If they don't believe me, I tell them that this or that herb is used to treat this or that. Then they see it is true.

I also tell them that my grandfather did not know everything. He used to refer some people to a bigger *sangoma*. They tell me that they do the same. Then we start to discuss things, and I can ask, 'Do you think you can treat all diseases, or are there some diseases you don't manage to cure?' Then they will tell you that they cannot cure this or that, things like tuberculosis, for example. Some of them refer patients with tuberculosis to hospital, but not all. Another thing they say they cannot manage is, when a child is 'dry' (dehydrated). They say that even when they try to 'make the cuts' (*a series of small incisions over the dieased area of the body*) there is no blood. They take the child to the hospital so that the Whites can put the blood back.

It is difficult to motivate the *sangoma* to co-operate with us. It must be done respectfully and slowly, through discussions. I know one who is co-operating with us well because we respected her. When we visited her for the first time, she refused to talk to us. She said that she did not want to talk to nurses but to doctors, because she is also a doctor. So then we visited her together with the Eye Doctor. She told us that she had problems with children who have diarrhoea, and asked what she could do for them. We showed her how to mix oral rehydration fluid. When we went to visit her again, she said, 'Give me your hand! That bottle you told me that I had to mix, it is working very nicely. I am even showing my other *sangoma*. I taught them how to mix it. They are now doing that system!'

'At first the traditional healer refused to talk to us nurses, and insisted on talking to an equal, a doctor. So we visited her with the Eye Doctor.'

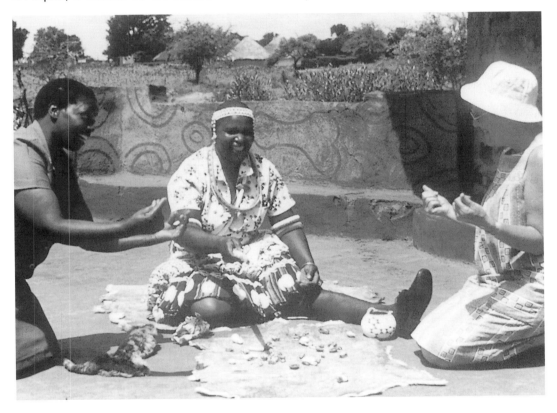

We said, 'Is it really working?' She said, 'It works very well! It gives us a good time to mix all the herbs for the child so that it will get well.' She has also stopped giving enemas to children with diarrhoea, which traditionally people used to do. She gives oral rehydration and advises the mother that when she is back home she must give the child some food, not soft porridge only, but everything.

2. Visiting homes in the community is not always easy

Care Group members may have difficulties when they visit highly educated families in their community, as these people may look down on them. The rich think, 'What is this poor woman coming to do here, what is she going to teach? We have everything here in this house.' But the good work done by the groups may convince the better-educated people that Care Groups have something to offer them, too – like the schoolteacher who learned from the Care Group how to treat her child's diarrhoea.

The schoolteacher is impressed

At the time of the cholera epidemic a Care Group who had just learned how to prepare oral rehydration fluid went round to teach all the people in their community. They covered the whole place, seeing that everybody could mix the fluid correctly. In one house they found a child that had diarrhoea. The Care Group member mixed oral rehydration fluid and gave it to the child. 'You must give it to the child each time it has a stool,' they explained to the mother, who was a teacher. The child recovered the same day. Later this lady teacher met a Care Group Motivator and told her, 'I did not believe that the Care Groups could be learning something which was really valuable. I used to ignore them. But now I know that the Care Groups are a good thing and I respect their work. I learned from the Care Group members how to prepare oral rehydration fluid, something I did not know about before. If I had the time I would like to join the group.'

Some religious beliefs and cultural differences can be a problem when we try to teach people about health. For example members of the Zionist church do not use any medicine, but heal with water, salt, coffee or tea. In their households, Care Group members feel they are not well accepted, and that people will in any case not do what they tell them. There are other people who use only traditional medicines and are ruled by their ancestors. Sometimes there are also taboos in the community, for example that one should not eat certain things, or that a person from outside is not allowed to enter a room where there is a very sick person.

Of course, it can happen that groups make mistakes when house visiting. I am thinking of one group which used to do their work very well, even when the Motivators did not visit them. They tried to organise things on their own. They kept on going round their village. There was just one thing where they went wrong, where they were misinterpreting the work of the Care Group. They used to say to the people, 'You must have a rubbish pit, you must have your yard clean, you must have a vegetable garden, etc.' They wanted to do their work well. The group wanted to be perfect. They didn't see that this is not a good way of motivating people. The word, 'You must' is very easy to say. We hear this word everywhere we go, at school, at the hospital and many other places. The people in the community hear it from the clinic nurse or from the Tribal Office. It is the way those who are powerful talk. So when Care Group members think they know more than the others in the community, and they feel a bit like nurses, they may start to talk like nurses.

3. Reaching all the members of a community

Divided communities

Many of the communities in the area were divided because of the forced resettlement that resulted from apartheid. When the 'homelands' were introduced in the 1970s, Tsonga communities which were settled in a Venda area were moved into Gazankulu, which was the 'homeland' designated for the Tsonga/Shangaan ethnic group. Before their removal, many people had been living near to Elim hospital or to the small town. There they had access to jobs and schools, and enjoyed a higher standard of living and better educational and health services than they did after they were forced to move.

In many places in our area there were two divisions. There were the people who had been staying there for a long time, and there were the people who came from somewhere else. We found that in such communities it was the people who came from other areas who were usually the first to join the Care Group. They were a bit better off and more educated than the people who had always been there. From the old part of the settlement very few joined, because they had other problems which were more urgent for them, like providing enough food for the family. That made people point fingers at each other. Some thought they were better than the others, and said the others were ignorant. This is always the problem in communities where there are people who have been staying there a long time and new people who have been brought in. These two groups don't mix after resettlement.

A divided community

In one community there were two parts. Section A was where the people who had always been there were living. In Section B there were people who had been resettled from a place near the main road. The people of A referred to Section B as 'Teakettle' – 'the place where the people were rich enough to have a tea kettle and drink tea'. More people in B could read and write. The first chairlady was from B. She was always active, and the Care Group members from her side were working well.

When we were still working on trachoma, and we started handing out eye ointment, we found that section A had too few members who had learned to examine eyes and apply ointment, although there was more trachoma there. The Motivators had to go to that side to help. In time, there came to be two groups, one in A and one in B. We wanted to get them together, so we organised a meeting together with the chief, for both sides to discuss.

At that meeting the people from B were sitting on one side, apart from the others. We did not know why they did not mix until we found out that the people from B felt they knew better than the ones from A, and the people from A were suspicious that B was getting more ointment. Finally, we arranged that the whole group would meet one time at A and the next time at B, and they would all have to come each time if they wanted to get ointment. After a while, the group decided that the arrangement was good and they should stay like that. However, this group is still on and off all the time, even after 25 years. The group falls apart whenever they are not actively doing something together like starting a communal garden or planning a crèche. Then they work very well together.

There was another problem for some groups in places where there had been resettlements. If the chairlady was from one side, the people from the other section were unhappy. They always wanted to support somebody from their own side. In some places, we never did manage to unite the two sections. In others we were more successful, but only after a lot of effort.

Division in the community was not always the fault of the women! There was one very big village where they had a lot of problems. People from five different places had been moved, together with their chiefs, to an area where there was already a chief. Now there were six of them, and every five years or so a different one was elected to be the chairman. When the Care Group members wanted to start organising themselves, the six chiefs were always quarrelling about where the group should meet, and the group could never get going. Finally, the women decided to go to the Tribal Office and tell them to stop quarrelling because they wanted to start to work. But the problem was still not solved. The strongest chief still wanted them to meet at his place at one end of the village, which meant that some members had to walk a long distance, so they stopped coming. Finally, the women divided into two groups, one at each end of the village.

Religious views can also divide communities. Once a group of women called us to come to their place, because they wanted to know what a Care Group was. We discovered that these women were 'Prayer Ladies' from their church. They listened to our explanations, and said, 'This is the work we would like to do.' We felt that they were very keen to start. We told them that the Care Group is open to everybody, and many other people came to join. We had meetings as usual. On one occasion, after giving a lecture we asked the group to think about it and make a role play or a health song. When the group had composed their songs, the members who had not been Prayer Ladies brought in a drum to accompany the singing. They beat the drum and danced with it. From that time on, when we went there, we did not find any of the original Prayer Ladies. They had disappeared, and they never came back. Only the other members were still there. We made investigations and found that the Prayer Ladies were against beating drums, dancing and wearing tribal dress. They did not want to do something together with the 'heathen'. They preferred European dress and new Christian names. But they never told us why they did not want to come any more.

'Are Care Groups really reaching the poorest in the community?'

Care Groups are open to each and every member of the community, rich or poor, educated or illiterate, men or women, regardless of religion. Because we wanted to include poor people in the Care Groups, we were discouraging when the groups were asking for a uniform. We suggested that they should rather use special head scarves, which everybody could afford.

But even so, are Care Groups really reaching the poorest in the community? It would be a good thing if we were reaching them, but I don't think we do, because when you see a very poor person, it is difficult to convince her to join a Care Group. She says, 'Oh, I am useless, I can't do such things.' They lack confidence, and we have to go closer to them to win them over. There are many who want to conceal their poverty. Also, the very poor people are often left out in their community and do not hear about what other people are doing. It might be something they would really like to join in with – but when they never hear how things could be improved, how can they ask for something they don't know about? In their experience, things never change for them – whatever they do.

There are some really poor Care Group members, but they are few. There are many poor people really in need of help who could benefit much from belonging to the Care Groups. Another thing with poor people is that they often have a fear of new ideas. They don't feel secure with something they don't know. They may also fear that if they get involved in something which is new to them, and find they do not like it, they will be stuck with it. Even Care Group members, who usually belong to the 'not-so-poor' section of their community, are often nervous about things they do not know.

I would like it if we could also get poor people to join the job creation projects. They are left out because you need money to start a project, and they do not have any money to put in. It has not yet come into the Care Group members' way of thinking that when there is a collection for the project, the very poor could maybe collect half as much as the others. But now some of the women have found their own good way. They work together as a group to earn some money which goes to the group's banking account, and they use that for starting a project. Then some poor people can be involved.

We are having some success. Many Care Groups are including poorer members of the community in their communal gardens. Another Care Group activity which was good for involving the poor is the peanut bulk-buying scheme, which was started during a period of drought. The Eye Doctor had met a farmer who was willing to sell peanuts at a low price to help the people. She introduced the Care Group Motivators to him, and he agreed to deal directly with us. The scheme is still going on and it works very well. The Care Groups buy big bags of peanuts, put them into small packets and sell them at a very cheap price. Then even two people can share a packet. When the peanuts come, they share, especially when they want to plant them to raise their own crop. Bulk-buying is a good way to reach the poor.

Places where it has been difficult to start Care Groups

There are some places where it has been more difficult to start a Care Group. For example, in some places where the church had been for a long time, most people were educated and did not want to listen to us Motivators who were only assistant nurses with little schooling. Also, such groups were not functioning well, because before, there had been leaders from the church, who did everything for them. They were not used to doing things for themselves.

One of the last places to join the Care Group Project was the community around the hospital. Most people staying there are working at the hospital. They thought they knew everything, and they were used to the missionaries doing things for them. One of our senior nurses was disturbed that her own community still did not have a Care Group, and she called for a meeting. She explained to the people that there were Care Groups everywhere except here. Why couldn't they start a Care Group? Then many stood up and volunteered. But when the time came that we called a meeting to discuss things, there were only a few, hardly 30. There were no young ones, there were old ladies only. Now, today, these old ladies are still going on. The group is collecting plastic bags, to clean up the area, and they use them to crotchet handbags. But they are getting older and older. Some have passed away. I think no new people are joining because the young ladies think they know enough – and if they do things, they want to be paid.

4. Working with and for the community

Many Care Group projects help the whole community – like making
concrete platforms around the water stand-pipes, so that puddles
do not form where mosquitoes can breed. In most places, the
community is happy about its Care Group and supports it. This is
especially the case where the members involve the community in
everything they are doing. We have experienced that these are the
groups that function best. The support of the people in the
community encourages them.

Now most Care Group members have understood what it means to
own their project, but there may be people in the community who
do not understand. Some think that Care Group members are very
lowly people and cannot do jobs needing special skills. For example
one Care Group was building a crèche, and was ready to be in
charge of the children. They were even training two members for
the job. But then there were some educated people who were
threatening them. They said that the Care Group mothers were not
educated, they couldn't be in charge of the children, and that they,
the educated, were going to apply for the job, so that they would
take care of the children and educate them. The Care Group
members who had been working very hard organising and building
the crèche would be pushed out just as the project began to show
fruit. That would have been very sad. But the Care Group members
stood together. They still own the crèche and work in it.

Communal gardens

An example of a Care Group activity which helps the whole
community is vegetable gardening. People who do not have time to
plant gardens themselves can buy fresh vegetables at a price they
can afford, and mothers who are not Care Group members can
also have a plot for planting. Even the Government realised that
communal gardens are a good thing to support. During the years
of drought in the early 1980s, the drought relief fund employed
poor people to clear the ground and erect fences. Those worst hit by
the drought could earn a little money, and more food was available.

However, it has happened that some groups forgot about their
purpose and wanted to have their communal vegetable gardens for
Care Group members only. It was a good lesson for us when we

found that Care Group members who were rejecting other community members in their communal garden had the problem that they themselves were rejected by the community, because the Care Group members were doing their own thing in their own small group. When these Care Group members went to visit other families in their community, they were not respected any more, because they were looked at as if they were only coming to 'shine' in these families.

In discussions in the group we asked ourselves, 'How are people feeling when we have our garden and we have vegetables and everything? And yet we are the ones who visit the families and tell them to eat vegetables which they don't have?' The group decided that it would be best to extend the garden and include other families who are not Care Group members – the poor, the disabled, and mothers of malnourished children. By growing their own vegetables, they can provide their children with better food. We see that communal gardens which also involve other people help the Care Group members to work well in their community. Because people are sharing in the Care Group garden, the group members are welcome in their homes and they thus have a better chance to give health education.

Today it makes me feel happy that there are now big community gardens which have Care Group members and 'non-Care-Group' members. The Agricultural Extension Officers come to demonstrate things like preparing seed beds and planting mealies, peanuts or *tindluwa* ('ground beans', which grow with the pods underground). These gardens are going on well. The ones where there are only Care Group members have more difficulties.

When there is trouble in a community, it affects the work

Something which makes the Care Groups stop working is when there is a bad thing happening in their community. We experienced a difficult situation at the time of the political unrest, before the elections for the 'New South Africa'. In places where people were killed for some cultural beliefs or other reasons, the Care Group members were scared to come to meetings. When a person has been killed, then all are sad and upset. Maybe that person was related to one of the Care Group members. The neighbours also feel like relatives, because they were used to that person. Then you cannot come from outside and have a meeting or start something in that community. You have first to sit and listen and sense it; you have nothing to say, because you can cause more trouble than there is already. That is something health care organisers are often not aware of, when they want to push us to do campaigns or whatever in such a community.

Vandalism: a new problem

Something that has started to happen recently, which is distressing the group members very much, is that unknown people are destroying structures for no known reason. Solar panels for the water pumps are stolen, taps at the water reservoir broken, buildings for the crèche vandalised. This is a bleeding wound for the group members, and we don't know how it can be healed. We hope the chiefs will be able to step in and take better care of Care Group property, which, in fact, is community property. But with so many people unemployed in present-day South Africa, problems like this are increasing.

Chapter 6

The joys and frustrations of being a Care Group Motivator

U nga tsutsumeli huku ni munyu

Don't chase a chicken with salt in your hand

Don't think the chicken is in the cooking-pot before you have caught it;
do things step by step

Chapter 6

The joys and frustrations of being a Care Group Motivator

1. Working in the community is different

We Care Group Motivators have many problems in our work which are our own secret, and we are shy of talking about them to our superiors. Yet I wish health care organisers and the other people directing us could know better how we feel and where we would like to get more help.

'We are on our own'

People from outside do not know the difficulties workers in the community can have. We are not protected, because we are on our own. We have to think and decide everything for ourselves. We must feel what to do, when to speak and when to keep quiet when people are very disturbed about something. We should be good listeners and good observers, in order to find out what people really want or need, because the people in the community usually do not say these things directly. If health workers in the community observe well, then they will know what people want. But even if they do know, they are often afraid to tell their superiors, so there is no feedback that can tell the doctors that something different should be done in that place. It was important for the beginning of the Care Group Project that we had a lot of confidence in the doctors in charge. They were willing to listen when we told them what we thought would be better for the community, and we knew they would not fire us.

In the community we have to watch what we do. We must discover our mistakes for ourselves. Sometimes I took a long time to realise that I was not doing the correct thing. It is a problem when you make a mistake which is difficult to change. I still think it was a good experience to struggle and to learn from what we did wrong, as long as we managed to correct it. But now we can share our experience with others, so they can get information from us, and do not have to repeat the same mistakes.

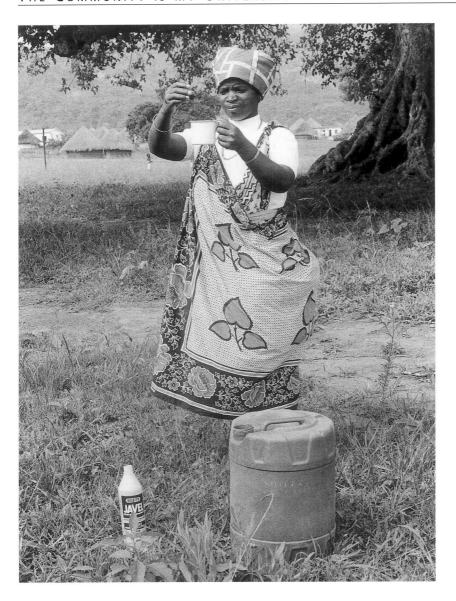

'We must take care not to confuse people. For example, we had to change our teaching about the amount of Javel fluid to use to chlorinate drinking water when the official recommendation changed from 5 drops to 20 drops – and people said, "Now you want to kill us." ' (Photo: E. Sutter)

'We must take care not to confuse people'

When people learn something which is not correct, it will take a long time to change what they do. Once you say something, people stick to it. We did sometimes have to change the methods we were teaching people. For instance, with chlorinating the drinking water we first used 5 drops of Javel water for 20 litres of water. People thought, 'Five drops is so little that it will not be poisonous, and it does not make the water smell bad.' But then a new official recommendation was made. The Community Health Doctor told us we must tell people to use 20 drops. And people said, 'Now you want to kill us.'

With oral rehydration fluid we decided ourselves to change the method. At first we had told people to measure the sugar with a tablespoon and the salt with a teaspoon. But we realised that they found it difficult to get the correct sizes of spoons, so we decided to tell them to use a teaspoon to measure both (8 teaspoons of sugar and 1 teaspoon of salt). The result was the same, but people got very confused, especially when other health workers came into the community and again used a different method.

As long as we Motivators were still new to the project, and were learning, we changed the groups between us very often, and the groups always had different Motivators. We thought this was a good way for Motivators to learn, forgetting that it might not be good for the groups. Then one group complained. They said this very straightforwardly one day when we were there:

> 'You people from Elim are confusing us. One day one person comes and says something, and another day another person comes and says a different thing. How do you think we can manage? Because when we did what you said, you said that you didn't say to do this – you were not the one who said that. Once we were told to take some money from the bank and buy some equipment for the crèche. Next time you said that money was not for equipment, it was for the building. It is the same with the people from the hospital coming all the time. We are tired of them. One day a nurse comes and gives an instruction. Next day the health inspector tells us something different. And our Community Health Worker again says a different thing – all about the same issue.'

Now we see to it that whenever possible, each Motivator is always in charge of the same groups. I have also noticed that a group is more active when there is always the same Motivator visiting them. They need time to get used to that person in order to trust her. This helps them to talk about things that are worrying them and inform us about community problems. This only happens after we have had many long discussions. It needs a good time.

'House visiting is useful, but it is not easy'

At one workshop for community health workers that I attended, we were told that the most important job in community health is to visit the homes, give health education, and give people advice when they are doing something wrong.

I agree that house visiting is useful, but it is not easy, because we are not always welcome, and we may even hurt people's feelings. People do not feel free when professionals visit their homes. I would not feel happy myself if the hospital superintendent were to come to my home without me knowing that he was coming! When people are still busy with jobs in their houses they are not ready for visitors they don't know. It shows that you don't respect their privacy when you just go into their homes. Traditionally we don't need to announce ourselves when we visit, because people visiting are mostly relatives and friends, and then it is normal to visit. When relatives visit and they see that some work has to be done, they just do the work together with the family. But when a person from the hospital comes, she will not take a broom and sweep the yard, or go and fetch water.

When a visitor comes who is not a relative, people don't know what she is coming for. Maybe the owner of the house has been busy with other work and has not yet managed to sweep. Then she will feel very embarrassed. If the visitor is from the hospital, she will think, 'The nurse is coming to look whether the house is clean', as everybody knows that the professionals always talk about cleanliness and food and all that.

People only begin to feel free when visitors come regularly, so they become used to them. Then they know that the visitor knows them well enough so when the house is not yet clean she does not think the owner of the house was sleeping late, but that she has been doing other work. It is important to train health workers and Care Group members to do house visiting in a good way. When groups are starting on a new task I visit them more often in order to do house visits with them. They should not make the same mistakes that we did when we started working with the communities, when people thought those visiting them were 'better people' who looked down on the lowly people in the community.

'You have to respect people'

It is important to know the culture. For example, I cannot start by calling somebody by her first name until I am used to her. I call her *Manani*, Mother, as a sign of respect for her. Some of the people also call me '*Manani* Maphorogo', which is a way of being respectful. For the elderly people it is good if one still shows them respect when one is visiting them, as in older times. People are now very much used to us because we know their customs and act according to their customs. If I enter the home of a Venda family and I see an old man or an old lady sitting there, I kneel. When I am there I do what everybody does and do all I am supposed to do. That is why people accept us.

You have to respect people. When you talk to somebody older than you and you say '*wena*' (the form used when addressing a child), that is not polite. Even if a woman is younger than you, but has a baby on her back, you must respect her, you should no longer say '*wen*a', you have to say '*n'wina*'.

2. Work in the community needs time to grow

'The doctor wanted to see things happening fast'

This problem of different feelings about time has been with us from the very beginning of the Care Group Project. When we started the Care Groups, the Eye Doctor was so busy with the patients in the hospital that she used to say things to us quickly. She thought that we understood what she said, but we did not understand. The things she talked about were new to us, and we could not follow her thoughts when we heard them only once. She also did not realise that I needed time to read the literature she gave me.

The Eye Doctor did not always realise what the problem was. If she wanted me to do something, she wanted it done *now*. But I felt I had to give it thought. I still wanted to find out how I could make it possible that what she was asking for would be successful. And she would observe me and think, 'Oh no, she is not interested'. And yet I was very interested – the only thing was that in my mind the idea was not yet ripe. Sometimes she said something I did not agree with or I did not understand, but I still kept it in my mind. And later on, when I realised there was now a need to do some of the things that I had thought were not possible before, I was ready to use the information, and I acted on it.

'When you hear something you have to give it time'

The European sense of time is different from ours. In our traditional culture, when you hear something you have to give it time. We don't act straight away. People who come from other areas act fast, and sometimes this means that mistakes can happen when rushing. In town it is different from the rural areas. Town people have adopted many things from European culture. I think if I went to work in a place in town, I would see things a bit differently, and I would have to learn a lot. When a person comes from town to work in the rural areas, he or she will say, 'Oh, it is useless with these rural people. They are just relaxing. They don't respond!' And if that community does not start straight away with the proposed project, the person from town gives up and does not go back to that group. But really the people are just taking their time. They want to look and see if it is possible. And when they are ready they ask, 'These people who promised to help – where are they? Now we are ready for them to come.'

Sometimes the Eye Doctor wanted me to go faster with the groups, to start something new when the group was still busy on something else. I told her that we would have to wait, because the Care Groups were not ready yet. I was glad that she used to listen to me and she waited. Not all doctors agree to do so. Most doctors coming from Europe stay only for a short time at our hospital. Then they are in a hurry to start a project in order to have results to take home.

There was a doctor from the tuberculosis ward who thought Care Groups could be useful to look after tuberculosis patients who had been discharged from hospital but still needed to be supervised for treatment. He wanted this to be started within one or two weeks. I thought, 'What shall I tell him?' I knew that if I said, 'Yes', the members would do it, but they would be handling a very serious thing, and if they were not clear about it, it could be dangerous. When we were not there with them, they would be responsible for the patient, who perhaps would not co-operate and therefore not get the correct treatment. People in the community cannot be asked to do something that was thought of overnight, even if it is something they eventually agree is a good idea.

One should have a good while to explain things and discuss them with the people until they understand. One should not rush and tell them what to do. Even if they can do it, they will not understand the aim of doing it. They will feel that they are doing it for somebody else, not for their own interest. People have to be sure that they really like a suggested activity, and understand how they should do it. A project does not last when the community is not with it. If there is something to be given to the community, some knowledge and skill, we need to give ourselves enough time to discuss it with the people and explain the purpose. In connection with tuberculosis, for example, people may already have their own cultural beliefs. And they need to know very well what tuberculosis is, if they are going to trace patients who have tuberculosis. They should know about the spread of the disease, and about its prevention. When they know all this, then they can go and discuss it with the contacts and the patients or with the other groups.

Any new activity in the community needs time. But this does not mean that the Care Groups cannot respond to new situations – even to emergencies. When there was the danger of a cholera epidemic, the doctors were worried that the community would be too slow to act. They thought the Care Group Motivators did not understand, so they were not pushing the groups fast enough. They thought we could tell the groups quickly, and the next day they would act. But it takes good discussions to make things happen. First, people must be able to recognise the emergency. Then they can think about it and can plan. If we just quickly inform the people about how dangerous the disease is, and give short instructions about prevention, it does not work. People will not understand enough in order to act on it. We need to talk about it many times. It will take maybe a week. One day is too short to convince the people.

Informing people about an emergency is more difficult in a new area where people don't know you. It needs people who know that place. There must be a person people trust, and once that person says something, the community will stand up. I would need to find out who are the people in a community who can make things happen. I would first approach them, and explain the situation to them very clearly. I would tell them that it is urgent. Then we could call mass meetings to discuss the issue. Once the key people understand the need, something can be started. We can start a survey next week, or start a campaign next week, if I can be given two days or three days to work full time in a community, just bringing awareness so that they will also see that it is urgent.

The problem of punctuality

People from Europe visiting the Care Groups often do not like it when the members are not yet there at the time of the meeting. They get nervous. 'Why can't these people be in time, why are some only arriving when the meeting is nearly over?' They forget that in rural areas there are only a few people who have a watch. People are used to measuring the time by the sun. This is why many have problems with keeping time.

There may be a group which will tell you to visit at such and such a time, and you will find them all there. There are other groups where they keep on reminding each other, even the same day, that they should be there at a certain time, and people are still missing. I understand why people are late. A mother coming back from fetching wood will first have to cook before going to the meeting. Some women are staying alone, and have to wait at home until the children come from school. The best time for the meeting needs to be discussed. Many women are very free at 3 o'clock. If we look at the time when they arrive, it is 3 o'clock. It also helps to make the members come on time if they know what we will be doing in the meeting, and they are interested. We have to inform them.

Sometimes a member arrives very late because she is leaving a very big problem behind. If you give her a bit of time, and do not let her feel guilty, she will start relating why she was late. It often happens to me that when it is time for me to leave, a woman who came very late comes to me and asks to see me privately. Then I cannot go home before I have heard what she is telling me. Of course, some people come late every time – that is another matter! But when it is not every time, then you are going to miss hearing about something which is serious if you are in a hurry to leave.

If we want the Care Group members to be in time we must also keep our appointments with them. When we tell the Care Group members that the meeting will be on a certain day, they will wait for us all day till sunset. But if no Motivator comes all afternoon, finally they will go home – and will not keep our next appointment because we have wasted their time. This means that you do not respect that for them time is also important. If a Motivator can't go to a meeting she must send a message and cancel the meeting. Care Groups lose interest when Motivators do not keep appointments. It damages work in the community and kills the spirit of the group. The Care Groups lose their trust in their Motivator. Whatever she will tell them, they will have their doubts. If you promise something to the community you must keep that promise.

3. What do people really think?

'Nurses don't know how patients feel'

The doctors think that if people are not using health services, it is because they don't know enough about them. But this is not the reason. It is because hospital or clinic nurses don't know how patients feel when being examined. They don't explain to the patient beforehand what is going to happen and what they will have to do. People feel ashamed when they just have to undress, because when they go to a traditional healer they are first told what treatment they will get to make them stronger so that witches cannot affect them. Then they undress with confidence, unlike at the clinic or hospital where they have to undress without explanation. Traditionally, undressing is part of the treatment, not of the examination. It was different in the eye hospital. There, we always explained beforehand what was going to happen.

In the same way the feelings of the people are not respected when nurses or health workers see a very sick patient. They think they have to force that person to go to hospital, but they do not give a good explanation why. They may even threaten with police, if the people don't agree. Now I know that one has to talk with the patient and the family, to know the reason why they do not want to go to hospital. Maybe they want first to be treated by the traditional doctor. We should respect the feelings of the patients and the wishes they may have. If we explain things to people politely they are more likely to agree to come to the hospital.

In the hospital, nurses address people in a way they would never do in their homes. They can call an old man by his first name, and the doctors do the same. This is very impolite. Doctors from Europe find it difficult to pronounce our names and often they are too much in a hurry. They take the easy way of calling people by their first names. This hurts the patients, and they feel uncomfortable and do not like the hospital. Sometimes we hear people complaining about nurses who come with the mobile child health clinic, 'Those people don't care, they don't talk to us.' There are some nurses people dislike, because of the way they do not talk to the mothers. They make them stand in a line, with their children undressed, then they just take the child and check its weight.

Spraying against mosquitoes: 'People would lock their houses ...'

Another example is that of the malaria control programme, which used to send teams to spray DDT in the houses to kill mosquitoes. They would announce that on a given day they would be at such and such a place to spray and that people should stay at home. But people would lock their houses and go away. They had a reason. The walls get white because of the spray. Sometimes they had painted the houses for Christmas and they looked nice, and then the sprayers came and then they looked ugly. This is the kind of thing that makes people oppose health interventions. If they had had enough information they would have understood why their houses had to be sprayed. As it was, they just thought that the spraying teams were careless and did not respect their property. I have heard of another spray which does not leave marks. I don't know why this was not used by the sprayers.

'Surveys disturb people'

When doctors and other outsiders are doing a survey, there is a lot of talk about it in the community. Surveys disturb people, even if many of them are useful and necessary. Doctors go into the community without knowing the community and without the people in the community knowing them. They use nurses and students to carry the questionnaires and to ask questions. When the people asking the questions do not know the culture of the people and how the people live, they may get misleading answers.

Long ago, when Care Groups had just started, some students from Johannesburg made a study of the Project. One of the questions was about the wealth of Care Group members and non-Care Group members. So the students asked the people if they had a radio, or dining room furniture, or things like that. I noticed that the students did not always get correct answers, because many people were thinking for a long time before giving an answer. They were looking to the sky and thinking, 'What does he want? Are they going to collect the furniture because I am behind on the hire purchase? It is better I say I have no furniture.'

That survey had actually been very well prepared. The Motivators had been going around the community, telling everybody what was going to happen. But still the people in the community did not trust the students. The chairlady of one of the groups told me that after the students had left the village her neighbour had come running to her and said, 'Don't be afraid of being arrested, I said nothing! These people asked if I knew Care Group members in the village, but I said I did not know any. I did not know if these people were from the police.'

Sometimes a student who needs to do a survey as part of a course goes into the community and starts work without explaining why he wants to do it. Then at the end of the survey that person disappears and the people keep waiting for the results. Sometimes the community members take a lot of trouble to tell the students everything, hoping that something will be done to solve the problems that exist in the community, only to find that it was for study purposes, and is not going to lead to any change. And maybe there is another survey, and again nothing is done. And maybe later people come to make a survey because they really want to change things, and the findings would have helped to do something useful, but people are no longer interested in saying all that they could say. They just say a few things in order to get rid of the interviewer, which is a pity. I think too many surveys have been done in our area. The people in the community are tired of them and they feel very unhappy.

The doctors and students who come to the hospital should start planning their surveys in good time, and they should start only after they have explained to the community why they want to do a particular survey, and planned it with them. They should also explain what they are going to do with the findings, and come back and tell the people about the results and discuss them. And it should not end there. Action should be taken according to the findings, because people have made the effort to answer all the questions, some of which may even be hurtful, for example when you ask a mother how many of her children have died.

When they are properly used, surveys can be useful

One survey that had really useful results was one in which we examined child nutrition with a medical student. This survey helped the people to see that it was important to have fresh vegetables, and after the survey they made a lot of small home gardens.

The results also led us Motivators to change our method of nutrition education. Before, we had just been telling the people which food is good, and how to prepare weaning food for the children by adding peanuts to the porridge. But when the survey showed us that children of Care Group mothers were not much better nourished than the children of non-Care Group families, we changed our method. We started cooking the food together with the mothers, and the children could try the porridge and the mothers could see that the children liked it. This encouraged the mothers to go on cooking the porridge at home, and they were teaching other mothers with young children.

Another result was that when that student became a doctor he chose to work in a rural area. In the end he became the superintendent of a hospital far away from us, and he was asking us to help him start Care Groups. Now there are many Care Groups where he stays. All that was the fruit of that nutrition survey!

Another survey that produced lasting results was one on trachoma, in an area where there were no Care Groups yet. A social worker prepared the people for the survey. He organised some community members to give health education to the people waiting to be examined during the survey. Every evening he asked the doctors for the results, and when he got some of the results after the survey was finished, he went back to report to the community about the findings. In this way he could motivate the people to do something about trachoma, and after three weeks a Care Group had started working in that place. I think this is the right way to do surveys, to report back to the community and to start acting on the problem together with the people.

4. Exploiting the Care Groups and their Motivators

'People do not like to be used'

Sometimes health services and others are using people for their own interests. If there is a special task to be done in a community and there is a shortage of staff, some doctors or clinic nurses remember that there is a Care Group, and they think they could use them for that task. But people do not like to be used. They always remark that the professionals earn money while they work for them without any pay. That is why we should discuss things carefully with the people first – then they may get interested, and feel they want to do what is being proposed.

Sometimes, doctors or development agencies want to try a new method or an idea they have, in a community that they have chosen themselves. It is then not something the people have asked for. If we try something that is inappropriate, people are disappointed. It is important to explain to people beforehand when something is being done as a trial.

It is difficult for someone who does not belong to the community to know what the people are really thinking about trials. When a doctor or other expert goes and introduces something new he wants to try, and later goes back to the community and asks if they are happy, people will say, 'Oh it is wonderful, we are so thankful for what you are doing for us.' They may actually be disappointed, and they may not like it – but the expert will never know the truth because people will not tell him. They don't want to disappoint him. Sometimes a doctor says something that he wants people to do, and if he does not observe well, and if he does not know the people, he will not discover that they are not with him. He will not see that they are not doing the things he was talking about. They will always say, 'Yes, there is no problem.' But they avoid the doctor.

'It is important to explain to people beforehand when something is being done as a trial'. At one time all the Care Groups were encouraged to plant Leucaena trees. In some areas it turned out that the trees did not grow well, and people were disappointed because their hopes of having a good supply of firewood were not fulfilled.
(Photo: C. IJsselmuiden)

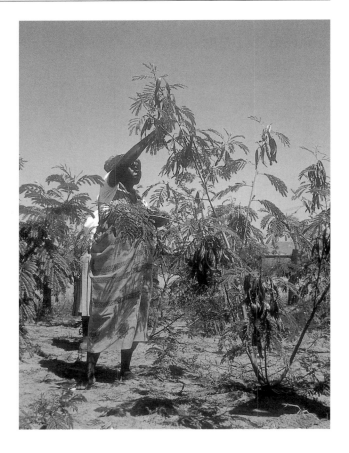

Last-minute projects and 'fly-by-night' experts

Sometimes you find that just before they go back to their home country, doctors want to show that they have been working very hard and that they have been helping people in the community. And we find that they are rushing to finish a survey, to get the results, to show back home that they have been working well and done a lot of things. Others make films to take back and show at home, but those films were only planned at the last hour, and they were staged, and do not show the real situation in the community that they are supposed to be recording. I don't know what they feel when they do such play-acting for two months and then they go. Is that a help for the community? Such surveys and activities are not fruitful – the ones that are only for the doctors' own success, and are published for their own sake and not to help the community to carry out a particular activity afterwards.

At one place where the Care Group was busy starting a communal vegetable garden, a development expert had the idea that the members could build a water reservoir with stones. He went to the group, and after a short discussion he started working with the members. People were carrying a lot of big stones, and then they made a big hole and were putting the stones in that hole, covering the walls of the hole. Then they bought cement and were filling the gaps between the stones. After they had finished, nothing happened. The expert disappeared, and there was no water to fill the reservoir. Now the Care Group members don't know what to do with that thing. I don't think it can hold water. It is a pity, because people spent so much energy, they were working in the sun, and working very hard, but they did not get any fruit from it. They were so disappointed, they even made a song about that reservoir. That is something to be careful of – to make a group work very hard, and at the end there is no result.

Care Group members working in other people's projects

People from outside who had heard about Care Groups often went to them first, wanting to grab their projects, by-passing the Care Group management team. Of course Care Group members could make a very useful contribution when they joined a project, because they were already trained and understood about things. This was good – but the Care Groups were often falling into the trap of joining all the organisations that came into the community, rather than going only where they were really interested.

Some people nowadays even pass remarks that the Care Groups are duplicating other people's work, forgetting that the Care Groups started with many activities long ago, and other organisations have only started now. We think they start on projects that Care Groups are already doing because they are ordered to do it like that by their supervisors or seniors. It can even happen that other organisations or community developers use Care Group members for their own purpose. They like to adopt Care Group members when starting a project. And then they tell everyone, 'We have done a good thing. We have trained these women.' Yet they were trained by us, the Care Group Motivators!

Chapter 7

Motivating and Mediating

Wonga n'hwari hi vutlhari, yi nga ti ku balekela yi haha
Follow the partridge cautiously, otherwise it will fly away
When working with somebody act wisely and kindly,
lest he run away

Chapter 7

Motivating and Mediating

When the Care Groups started, Community Health was not a high priority of the Health Services. Hospitals did support the groups as part of their outreach programmes. However, just as the attempts of doctors to move into the community had been misunderstood by their colleagues, the work of the Care Group Motivators and the groups was often misunderstood by the hospital-based staff. As Selina Maphorogo so often insists, 'Working in the community is different.' The problem of 'serving two masters' has dogged the Care Group Motivators from the beginning.

Care Group Motivators have many years of experience in working for health in the community, and many of them have had a lot of specialised training. However, they are generally still employed by the Health Services, and their official status is still that of assistant nurses, because their formal training places them at that level in the hierarchy.

When the Health Services became more concerned about outreach, Community Health Workers (CHWs) were introduced. They were at the same level in the hospital hierarchy as the Care Group Motivators, and were expected to work in the community – indeed, in the 1990s the superintendent of one of the hospitals even decided that as there were too few Motivators, CHWs should take over the Care Groups. However, their training and experience were not always appropriate for this type of community work.

Another change since the Care Groups started is that there are more people working in the village communities, whose aims and ambitions often overlap. Since Care Groups are now involved in so many aspects of community development, the Care Group Motivator often has to mediate not only between the community and the Health Services, but also between organisations and individuals from outside, to try to ensure that the activities really benefit the community.

1. Between the hospital and the community

The hospital's medical superintendent and senior community health nursing staff recognise the value of the Care Groups, but they would not be able to run the Project, as nurses are not trained in community development or in running job-creating projects. There are still some who do not understand that our Motivators do more than just talk about health. This creates misunderstandings, but this can be corrected.

One thing which disturbs all the grass-roots workers – both Care Group Motivators and CHWs – is that we are between the hospital and the community. We have to follow the instructions of our supervisors at the hospital and at the same time to try to do what the community wants. As Motivators, we work together with the Top Executive of the Care Group association. They are our seniors for the things concerning the community. We should ask them how they would like us to help and what we should do. But when the health team wants to make a vaccination campaign, our supervisors at the hospital don't call for a meeting with us to discuss it; they just give orders that we must work on the campaign. We are not given a chance to cancel our appointments with the Care Groups, and the groups may get discouraged, and may not attend the meeting the next time. Motivators and CHWs need to be given good information about what they should share with the community, and when they will have to take part in activities organised by the Health Services.

Working together to meet the community's needs

There are some projects where we have achieved good co-operation. For example, since we have a nutrition unit at the hospital, and we work well together with the doctor of the children's ward, we have started a new method of involving the Care Groups. When the malnourished children are discharged from hospital, we refer them to the Motivator who is going to the community the child comes from, who then talks to the Care Group members and asks them to advise and help the child's mother. And when mothers are having problems in getting food, the Care Group involves them in their garden.

The Care Groups themselves can suggest ways in which they could co-operate with the Health Services, so that together they could meet the needs of the whole community as well as those of individuals. This is a way of putting Primary Health Care into practice with the people themselves. One Top Executive suggests how co-operation between Care Group members and the Community Health Workers (CHWs) could function:

'A CHW is supposed to go out on certain days to visit the people. But often she has work in the clinic and has not enough time to visit the families, so she will never manage to cover the whole area. With the help of the Care Group she can manage it. We come together and inform the CHW what is happening at each corner in the community. And when we see a problem we tell her and she can go and see. That is where we need each other. If there is no CHW, we go to the clinic to tell the nurse about a problem we meet, or we accompany the patient to the clinic.'

The doctor of the children's ward sends mothers of malnourished children to learn how to cook weaning food. This is an example of the way the members of the hospital Health Team and the Care Groups can work together. (Photo: M.- A. Gneist)

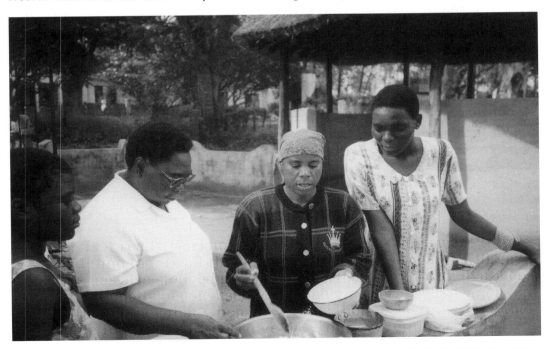

Nurses do not always appreciate what the Care Groups can do

Nurses often work with Care Group members, during vaccination campaigns or when we invite them to teach the groups something special of which we have no knowledge. Some nurses, who do not know what Care Groups are, and that the members have a lot of skills and knowledge, are not aware that they should share the tasks with them. They often think that nurses' regulations do not allow them to let Care Group members do certain tasks. For example, during one polio vaccination campaign doctors, nurses, motivators and Care Group members were all working together as one team. Later, a nurse joined us for the first time. She did not know how the Care Groups work, and she strictly followed the nursing regulations. She did not want the members to give vaccination drops. She stopped a mother from giving the drops, asking her, 'What do you know about vaccination? You are not trained as a nurse. You can line up the people for me.'

'Care Group mothers showed that they can do very good work when they treated trachoma and improved personal hygiene. People used the little water they had to wash their hands and faces.' A practical demonstration during a house visit. (Photo: E. Sutter)

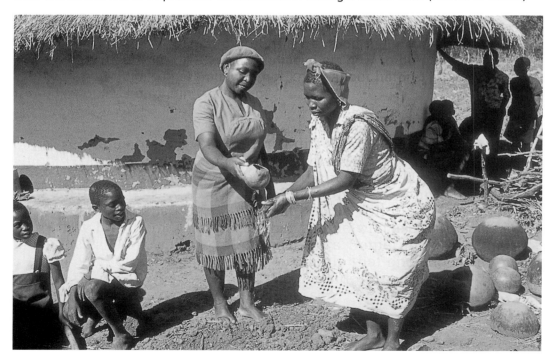

The Care Group mothers felt very bad, because they knew they could give the vaccination correctly. They were also not happy because the nurse said this in front of all the people, so that the community might think that Care Group members were not well trained. We know that the Care Group members could work very well when the health team explained to them carefully how to do it and supervised them. There are things any person can manage. A Care Group member can count the three drops for polio vaccination, and then she can assist in a polio vaccination campaign. One does not need to go to University for that!

The Care Group mothers showed that they can do very good work when they treated trachoma, and improved personal hygiene and the standard of living in their community. Wherever we go, we find that every house is very clean. The utensils are clean, and the children are clean. You don't need to study for that.

2. Community Health Workers or Care Group Motivators?

The Care Group Motivators are all trained as assistant nurses, and at the beginning, the people in the community sometimes saw us as being like nurses. Later, when Care Groups were already functioning well, Community Health Workers (CHW) were appointed to work in the community.

The first CHWs trained in Gazankulu were women chosen by the community. The requirement was that they should have been educated up to Standard 6, that is, they had 8 years' primary schooling. Some of them had been Care Group members for a long time, and were suggested for training by their Care Groups. They were trained at a Health Centre, and their practical work was done mostly in the community. We Care Group Motivators helped with the training. These CHWs all knew what Care Groups were, and after training they worked very well hand-in-hand with the Care Group.

Later, there was a new regulation, that CHWs must have 'matric', the school-leaving certificate obtained after 12 years' primary and secondary schooling. They were then trained in the hospital by the nursing tutors, and had little experience of working in the community. Most were not chosen by the community. They were young girls who often had no interest in community work and regarded it simply as a job. These hospital-trained CHWs were then allocated to take care of the Care Groups in the communities where they worked. This also happened in our Health Ward. The Motivators were no longer supposed to go to the Care Groups in places where there was a CHW. But these young CHWs did not have the skills for guiding the groups, or for community development, and the Care Groups complained that they were being neglected.

An additional problem was that even if the CHWs wanted to respond to the needs of the community, they did not feel free to do so. Those responsible for the health services did not trust the CHWs and felt that a nurse should supervise them. If a CHW was told to help at the clinic, she had to go – she was afraid to tell the nurse that she had other things to do in the community, like attending a Care Group meeting. The Care Group Motivators could have shared their knowledge and skills with the CHWs, but they had no chance to do so, because training was supposed to be done by a higher-ranking person.

The ideal Community Health Worker

The people in the community are very clear about what type of a person a CHW should be and what she should do. They want a woman with experience who they can respect. This is how some Top Executive members see the problem:

'We see the Community Health Worker as a child of the Care Groups, because often she has been a Care Group member herself and was chosen from the Care Group. But sometimes, when she has been trained for her new job, she forgets that we should still work together. She is given orders by the Health Office to do this and that. Sometimes, when she is supposed to attend a meeting with the Care Group she suddenly gets instructions from the Health Office to do something else. We would like to sit together with her and discuss together. When she meets with the people at the grass roots – the Care Group and the community – she can find out what the community needs.

'The nurse at the clinic is not at the same level as the community, and is not in such a good position to bring knowledge right to the grass roots. The CHW, who is from the same community, could be even better than the nurse at doing Primary Health Care in the community. But often what the CHWs do is aimed at satisfying the Health Office; they are working for the matrons, not for the community.'

3. Working together for community health and development

The 'Professionals'

Care Group Motivators and CHWs are at a similar level of training. Other community workers have a higher education. They are what I call 'professionals'. They help by doing new things with the groups. This is very good, and is useful to the groups and to us as Motivators. We can learn together with the groups and can then use the new methods elsewhere. In this way, Care Groups have learned how to build toilets and mud stoves; they have learned good methods of cooking and child care, and many other things. But it needs good planning, and working together from both sides, the Motivators and the specialists. Sometimes one or the other of us does not manage so well, especially when the specialists have not enough experience of working with the people in the community, and do not realise that we could help them.

Outsiders do not always understand

Professionals who come to work in the community, for example doctors and nurses, agricultural extension officers, or representatives of development organisations, are mostly outsiders, and do not have experience of how the community members live and feel. We Care Group Motivators could be of good assistance to them. We are mixing with the people the whole day, sharing each other's problems. As we are on the same level as the people in the community we know about the people's culture, their needs, what is disturbing them and what they want.

But because we are 'only' assistant nurses and are on the lowest rank of health workers, we are often not considered, even if we have more experience than people from outside. Misunderstandings can happen which could have been prevented or solved through discussions and understanding. Our experience has been that, if we plan together and work hand in hand together, then things go well. There have been many times when people from outside were helping and supporting us, but I also want to talk about others which caused problems for us and the community. It is not to point fingers, but to improve our work together.

Many people and organisations who came into the community did not have the idea of looking at what was already happening, and building on what was there already. Also the different project leaders were never sitting down to plan together. They didn't know each other, and they didn't know who knew what in that community. The cars just met, but nobody knew who was doing what.

When many organisations start to work in the villages, people get confused, because they are not clear about their aims. Apart from that, when people who do not know the culture and the local situation go into a community and start work they may cause problems that make it harder to achieve their aims. For example, they may not realise that the support of the chief is important if a project is to succeed. The story of the outside project that tried to introduce mud stoves to a village without consulting the chief is a good example.

Mud stoves are excellent – in the right place

Some people from an outside development organisation once came to make a mud stove as an example. They chose to make it at the chief's place in one of the communities, though they had not discussed it with him before. It was also not an appropriate place to build a mud stove. When these people got to the chief's house he was not at home, only his wife. She knew nothing about people coming to build a stove, but she was afraid to say 'No'. In the evening when the chief came home, he was furious to see that stove in his house. He destroyed it before it could be used, and no one could go and see it.

Later, the Care Group members thought of making a mud stove at the clinic for the waiting mothers so that they could use it, and learn how to build one in their homes. There was a nice *rondavel* which was donated by the local business man. But when the chief heard about this stove, he went off to the clinic and told the Care Group mothers that he did not want to see a mud stove there. He told them to remove it, and they had no choice but to obey. The chief had been offended when those people from outside came to his house without making an appointment and built that stove he did not want. He was now against any mud stove in his community.

Another project that did more harm than good was one for building toilets with the Care Group members. This would have been a very good project, but the development worker concerned did not take the trouble to learn about the local situation beforehand. He tried to separate the people from the chief. He did not know that this particular chief was a very helpful one, who was working very much hand-in-hand with the Care Group, and supported them in whatever they would like to do. It was this chief who worked with the people when the group organised a firewood plantation. He used to have a good way of discussing things, but now, since the toilet project, he has changed his attitude. Nowadays, if he wants the group to do something he just tells them, he no longer discusses it. The Care Group is now confused. Until today, the group has not managed to come back exactly to what it was before – and the toilet project has stopped.

The need for co-operation is greater than ever

When we started with the Care Groups there were few things women could join. There were the Prayer Women from the church, a few women's clubs and some literacy classes. Other organisations came to start their own projects later, when Care Groups were already everywhere in Gazankulu. Nowadays, there are many different people who work in the community. There are people working with health or with community development, such as doctors, health inspectors, matrons, nurses, Care Group Motivators, agricultural extension officers, literacy educators, teachers or development workers. They are all community workers, no matter what profession they have, and they should co-operate, to help the community reach its aims. As Care Group Motivators we have to do with all of them.

It is always nice when community workers organise meetings to plan together, or organise joint functions. This avoids misunderstandings, because the community sees that we are united and help each other. It gives room for better communication, and no one feels superior or junior or looks down on community members and other community workers. People help each other when there is a need and consider what each one is doing. We are not going to point fingers when things go wrong, but work towards solving the problems and give each other advice. Then the community is helped to reach its goal, and we will be happy when the community has trust in all of us. There is a proverb saying, '*Ritiho rin'we a ri nusi hove.*' This means, 'One alone cannot manage, but together we can win.'

But sometimes we have problems when working together. Maybe the Motivators and a development worker want to work with the same Care Group. We do health discussions; he is building toilets. This can be a good thing. But we must agree on the dates for meeting with the group – when we arrived for an appointment with the Care Group to cook weaning porridge and found the development worker already there, doing something else with them, it was bad planning! We should have worked as a team together. We tried to solve the problem and co-operate with him, but it did not help. Each party kept on doing things separately.

There is also a danger that when people do not find out what is already going on that they will waste their efforts. For example, there were some occupational therapy students who wanted to start a project in one of the communities where there was a Health Centre. There was a Care Group in the same place, which was already doing a lot of things – including sewing wonder boxes. The occupational therapists did not contact the Care Group, but went directly to the Health Centre, and they got another group of women together. Some of them were Care Group members. They said, 'We are going to teach you how to make a wonder box.' But the Care Group members already knew how to make wonder boxes! Through discussing together the problem could be solved, and the students came to understand that it is best to work with the Care Groups, not to start something which will flop when they are gone. That project now works very well.

'Everyone has their special skills'

Just as the Care Groups and the Health Services can achieve more by co-operating, projects for community development will be more effective if we work together with other people like water and sanitation experts or the Agricultural Extension Officers (AEOs). However, they have to be ready to co-operate with us. For a long time we kept on having difficulties with the AEOs. When they had finished their studies they were allocated to communities. They did not find out what was already going on in their villages. In one village where the Care Group already had a garden they just looked at the place quickly and then started another garden on the other side. The Care Group members were struggling with their garden, because they did not have enough money, and had to pay back the money they had borrowed from the revolving loan fund. The others had money from the Agriculture Department, and they could hire people to work in their garden. The AEOs worked very hard on their own garden, and neglected the Care Group one. It became a competition between the gardens. And as the people working in the Government garden were earning wages, some Care Group members left their own garden and went to work in the other one.

We struggled a lot to discuss matters with the AEOs. The Care Group members had some skills, which they had got from the Valley Trust (Chap.2, p. 77), but not enough for everything they wanted to do in their garden. We encouraged the two groups to come together and network to produce something for the community, instead of confusing the people and starting to point fingers at each other. We were successful, and now we work very well together and both sides are happy and are learning from each other. People will trust community workers, when they see that we all work together and assist each other.

Another problem we had was that when we started with the deep trenching method for the communal vegetable gardens, which we had learned from the Valley Trust, the Department of Agriculture did not like it. They did not know the method themselves, and in some areas they even told the Care Groups to stop using it. They only began to co-operate with us when there was a new Director of Agriculture, who went himself to the Valley Trust to see what they were doing there, and saw that it was a good method.

A good example of co-operation is the story we told in Chapter 4, about the women in Y who had a big quarrel over their communal garden. The AEOs could not manage to get the quarrelling women together. But when we went with them to have discussions with the group, we managed to sort out the problem. They needed us because we have learned a lot about organising groups to work together. We needed them because, though we have learned something about farming, we can't tell anybody about cultivating peanuts or what they should do when the mealies turn yellow. As long as we understand that everyone has their special skills, co-operation is easy.

Chapter 8

Looking back and looking forward:

experience from the past and dreams for the future

Masungulo lamanene ya vevukisa ntirho

Well begun is half done

Chapter 8

Looking back and looking forward:

experience from the past and dreams for the future

1. 'The Care Groups are my University'

When I look back I can say that I gained a lot since starting with Care Groups. When I compare myself before my appointment as a Care Group Motivator and now, I see two different pictures. Before, I did not know how to solve problems. I was very shy even to say good things. During meetings no one could hear my voice except when I was asked to say something. I just did the things I was expected to do or was asked to do by my seniors.

Now I am thinking for myself what I should do. In the community I learned to work with others. I managed to find a better way of communicating, and to know the correct behaviour, respecting people. Now I can stand in front of people, listen to them and observe, and then discuss with them what they want to do. When there is something I don't know I can say so, and I am ready to accept corrections.

I learned a lot at Manchester University and in London. Many people have assisted and taught me, and organised things so that I could attend courses. But most of the things I know, I learned from the people themselves. Care Groups are my University. I feel proud of the way I learned, because I was trying to get things by myself, and I was happy to find that the people in the community liked what we were doing. Finding out things for yourself is not like hearing it from other people who have already done it. If you have your own experience you understand why you do something and you will not forget. Since I started to read books and understand what I am reading I found that many of the things we did were quite correct, and there were only a few things which were not right.

I am now able to share my experience with others. I have been invited to many places, for example to Ghana where a women's group wanted to exchange ideas with us, or to Switzerland, where I took part as a facilitator in a course for doctors and nurses in the

Swiss Tropical Institute. But the greatest encouragement for me
was being nominated as South African Woman of the Year 1996.
Now at last my own country has given official recognition that the
Care Groups are important for rural development.

Much of what I say for myself is the same for everyone in the
Care Group Project. We all gained in strength and learned to stand
up for what is right. Motivators learned to work with the people,
not just for the people. Care Group members gained confidence,
and the groups have become platforms for development in their
communities. Care Groups are now organising themselves and are
no longer so dependent on the hospital and the Motivators. But the
path to success has been too long, because of mistakes we made
while we were learning.

Now it is different. There are many health and development projects
in South Africa and in other countries, and people can exchange
experiences. Many organisations in our area are learning from our
style of working in groups and the way we are communicating
with villagers. We share with them what we learned from the
things we did wrong, so that they will not make the same mistakes.
In this last chapter I want to put some of these lessons in writing,
to help others who would like to start something like Care Groups,
so that they will not fall into the same traps that we did.

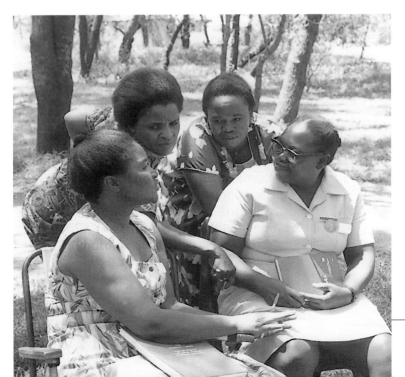

Sharing experiences
with leaders of other
development projects
at a community
health workshop.
(Photo: E. Sutter)

2. Lessons from experience

This is a list of some things that I think we did wrong. It is worth discussing them and finding ways to do better:

- We started community work without being trained for the job.

- Some Motivators who were employed by the Project were not carefully chosen and were not the right persons for this particular job.

- When other Health Wards joined the Project their Motivators were trained at Elim, not at the place they were going to work.

- Care Groups were mothered too much by the Motivators and for too long. This made the groups dependent.

- We failed to communicate well with the hospital's public health team and with other people acting in the community like agriculture and community development organisations.
  This was confusing for the Care Groups.

'If I could start again, training would be my first priority'

When we started with the Care Groups we had no experience. We didn't know exactly what we wanted, and we made a lot of mistakes. We were the only ones who went into the community to work on health with the people, so there was no place which had already done something like the Care Groups where we could ask for information. The doctors tried to help us with refresher courses, and weekly meetings to discuss our problems, and some of the nurses and matrons also tried to help us. But at the beginning of the project, all of us were still learning, and the Eye Doctor did not know what to train us for. On the whole, we had to 'learn by doing'. We just went out to the people and taught them as we thought it was the way to do it. We were lucky that we started with trachoma, a disease people knew about. From there we could go on. But the problem was that once trachoma was no longer so important, we did not have enough new things to give to the groups. I could see with some Care Groups which were flopping that it was not because they were not interested, but because we didn't have anything new to give to them.

I have already told the story of how I did succeed in learning on my own, with the help of the people in the villages. But I still feel I miss having had training before I started work in the community. Even after I have attended many courses and workshops, a feeling of insecurity remains with me. This is why I would no longer send Motivators into the community without any training. If I could start again, training would be my first priority.

How I would like to see Care Group Motivators being trained

Motivators should be trained in the community
During all the courses I enjoyed I found that my best teachers were those who had worked in the communities themselves. I have also seen that the results of the first training course for CHWs, which was held at a rural health centre, had better results than later courses that were in the hospital. A person who is going to work in the community should be trained in the community, not in the hospital. If possible, she should be trained in the area where she is going to work. Then she will know how to use the local resources and how to build on what the people know and have already. She will know what a Care Group is and what other organisations have done already in the same place, so she can avoid duplicating the same activities. When she starts work on her own, she will already know what type of community she is going to serve and what problems people have. The other community workers will already know her and will help her whenever she needs support.

Practical training in the community is the most important part of the course. But besides this, the Motivator should learn other things like adult education and training skills (e.g. role playing and story-telling in health education), needs assessment, and project planning and evaluation. It is always good for group and project leaders to know something about project administration, for instance about simple bookkeeping so they can help the groups to handle their money. Motivators should also be trained in running meetings and forming committees and in good ways of communication, and they should know how to write reports for those who assist the groups financially.

At the end of such a training course the Motivator will be ready to start, and will not fall into the same traps as we did, when we were pushed into the community without knowing what to do and made a lot of unnecessary mistakes.

Motivators should know about health – in theory and practice
Since Care Groups work in the field of health, the Motivator must have a good knowledge of the important local health problems. She should know how to prevent common diseases and how to promote good health according to the needs of an individual community. During the course, she should also learn where she can go for help when she has a problem she cannot solve, and it should be made clear that she must never be shy about asking for assistance when she needs it.

Supervisors often believe that the job of a health educator or a Motivator is only to talk and to give health education, so she does not need practical skills. But the community expects her to be able to deal with emergencies like accidents, or women going into labour when there is no nurse around. What do people think after an unexpected birth, when someone employed as a health worker is not allowed to separate the baby from the placenta, while an elderly woman does it with dirty scissors? CHWs and Care Group Motivators should have basic knowledge about maternal care and first aid in case of emergencies. And they should know how urgent a case is and whether the patient should be taken to the clinic.

Refresher courses and further training
As community workers we often felt we had been left alone with our problems. It is therefore important that Motivators get regular follow-up in refresher courses. This also gives them a chance to share good and bad experiences with other Motivators and to see that all have similar worries. The courses provide a good opportunity for attitude and leadership training. In role-playing and open discussions, Motivators are made aware that we are all the same, and that we should help each other. This includes being ready to accept being told by Care Group members when there is something we are doing wrong, and correcting ourselves. We should not get cross, because they are right to tell us. Myself, I am happy when Care Group members are not shy, because it helps us in our work.

Refresher courses can remind Motivators that community workers should not be selfish but should share what they know with the Care Group members. We need to be aware that we all tend to want to show people that we are clever. This makes us talk in a way that makes Care Group members feel ignorant. It is important for Motivators to learn how to choose things to talk about which the people can understand, not things which are too much above them.

As Care Group Motivators, we have already learned a lot about problem-solving with the groups. This is much easier than to solve problems between ourselves! A special effort should be made to learn to work as a team. It would help us to grow in strength and would benefit the Project.

Training should not only be within the Care Group Project. Future leaders should do more to encourage the Motivators to attend short courses elsewhere on topics which are useful for their work with the groups, where they will also see other teaching methods and learn about other people's views. I have been lucky in having a chance to go to other areas to see what other people are doing, so I could get new ideas. Many of the other Motivators have been too shy about going away from home, so they missed important experiences outside their local situation.

Further training is vital. Motivators at a book-keeping course. (Photo: E. Sutter)

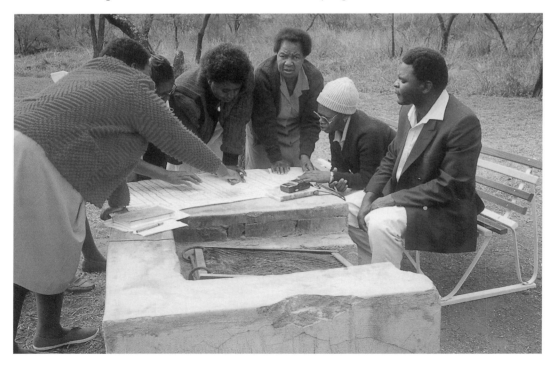

The selection of community workers

It is not everybody who can become a good community worker, however well she is trained. She must be a person people can trust. They must feel free to share their worries with her and ask her for advice. Mothers would not like to discuss family matters with a young, unmarried girl. It is only for questions outside family life, where expert knowledge is needed, for example in agriculture or village technology, that a young person with these special skills would be accepted. In our culture, we would only ask for advice on family matters from other married women who have their own experience with husbands and children. In community work, we also need time to make friends with the people we work with. If we train a young girl she might get married and leave the community with her husband before people have had a chance to get used to her.

A Motivator must have her heart in the work, and not just join the project because she wants a job. If she does, when she has difficulties with a group she may just say, 'I don't mind whether you come to the meeting or not. I can go back to the work in the hospital, and I still earn my salary. I have no problem. I have water at home and I have food.' Such a person goes to the groups as a superior. She expects people to say 'Yes' to her about everything she says. Especially if she was trained in the hospital, she would really prefer to stay in the hospital and not work in the community.

There is also the question of education. A Motivator must be able to read and write, and be educated at least up to Standard 6. It is true that we need people in our team who have something new to contribute, and we may find them among those with more education. But if a young woman has a Standard 10 school certificate, she may get a chance to do nursing training, and leave after a short time. There is also the problem that a better-educated person may not be ready to listen to and respect the community members. Of course, this does not apply to better-educated people only – when anybody joins the Project we need to see what their attitude is. But I always say we should not be too quick to say someone is not fit. We might be losing a good person who might still learn. I know from my own experience how long it can take.

The perfect Motivator

I have a picture in my mind of a perfect Care Group Motivator. She (or he) has been chosen by the community according to their expectations. She is somebody who is committed and willing, who knows how to behave politely, and who can communicate well with the community members and likes working with the community. She also has other skills, and is ready to keep on learning. Finally, she (or he) must be a good leader for the group – one who does not sit high up on a chair while the group members sit on the ground, but sits down with them to show that they all are the same and nobody is superior, and that they all help each other.

One day we discussed with the Top Executive and other Care Group members what kind of Motivator they would like to work with. This was what they had to say:

> 'At some hospitals they allocate just anybody who wants to be a Care Group Motivator to work with us. They just say, "Come and work for Care Groups." They must work for Care Groups, and yet they don't know what they are supposed to do. This is not fair. People should know what a Care Group is. The hospital should let us employ our own workers. When the Health Office employs people they want educated people, those who have "matric". When it comes to Care Groups, the Project has no money to employ people with a higher education who want a big salary. If we were allowed to employ whoever we wanted, we would choose people who know the Project and who have the skills needed.'

3. Passing on what we have learned

Starting community projects

Since people have got to know about the way we are working with the Care Groups, it often happens that people wanting to start a project in our area come and discuss it with us. I am always glad when people want to know which projects are already in the community – unlike some people who just come in and start.

When we start something at a place we don't know, we first go to people who are trusted by the community there, and discuss it with them. We know we have to depend on people who are already there – it must not be us going to the community first, and starting something. This is a very clear thing for me. A doctor who was interested in helping us with the Care Groups once said, 'You know, I depend on you, because I don`t know the situation, and people don't know me. I do not know what people want to learn or what they want to know.' This is a good attitude when starting a new thing.

Encouraging groups to be independent

It is better not to be with the groups all the time. In some groups there are powerful women who know how to run things. We see now that in places where we did not go very often, the Care Groups gained confidence that they could do things by themselves. They met on their own, without us. If groups always wait for a Motivator to come, it prevents them from becoming self-reliant and it can delay their work, because if we make an appointment and fail to go or can't reach the place because of rain, or a puncture, they sit and wait for the Motivators to arrive, and if we are not there they go back home.

In our area, we waited a long time before we started to form an association of Care Groups. Now, I think that if people want to start Care Groups I would advise them to guide the groups from the start towards taking the step of forming an association as soon as they are ready for it.

Sometimes, Care Groups tend to fall into the trap of joining in with just any project or activity that comes into their community, without first looking carefully at whether they really want it. To avoid this, it is important for groups to be very clear from the start about how they want to function and what their aim is.

Making sure that the approach is right for each place

People who want to start Care Groups often ask if they can come to observe groups that are already working. This is a good idea as a start, but then they have to go back and look at the situation in their own place, and adapt the work to it. It is also important that when people come to look at Care Groups and discuss how to start a project of their own, it should not be only the future Motivators who come, but also other people from the hospital's public health team, like nurses and health inspectors. Then everybody will be informed about the project from the start. That should help the new Care Group project to avoid the kind of communication problems we experienced.

People in other places should not just imitate the groups in our area. When one hospital very far away wanted us to train Motivators for them here at Elim, I did not think it was a good idea. Their problems are not the same as the problems we have in our area. I said it would be better for them to invite some Motivators from Elim to come to them and go round their communities with them. Then they could all discuss things together and find a way to overcome the problems.

Sometimes people ask me if Care Groups would also work in other countries, or in a town. I have seen community projects very like ours in rural areas in other countries, for example in Ghana and in Mozambique. There they work well. I have no experience with towns. I believe Care Groups could be established in towns, but it would be difficult because in a town too many cultures are mixed, and there are too many different interests. Also, there are usually more educated people in a town, and educated people often think they know everything already and do not need something like Care Groups.

For Care Groups to work successfully, people must have something in common – a common need on which they want to act. Then a group might be started by the people themselves. For example, maybe one could start a group in a town with mothers attending the Child Health Clinic. *(During times of political unrest under the Apartheid Government, mothers in the townships did unite, in an attempt to prevent police from arresting their children and throwing them into jail. E.S.)*

4. Dreams today – reality tomorrow?

A united health team, with members who listen to each other and to the community

Today, we have Community Health Teams. It is important that the people in the community see that we as a Health Team are all one: the doctors, the nurses, the Care Group Motivators and Care Group members. Then the people will trust us. I saw this happening once, during a polio vaccination campaign. There we were all working together. It was a wonderful day – I was so happy! The Care Group members gave the polio vaccination, the three drops in the child's mouth. All the children were weighed and examined. The ophthalmic nurses looked at the children's eyes, and the physiotherapists checked the children for disabilities and gave advice. Care Group members also cooked weaning food. Everybody was happy seeing us helping the community.

Unfortunately, this ideal does not always work. Often we fail to communicate well within the Health Team, even though we have a common office for this purpose. Then we go to the villages with different messages, and the people complain that we from the hospital are confusing them.

We should not be shy about sharing our knowledge with each other in the Health Team. We all have different tasks and skills. Doctors and nurses know all about health, and the Care Group Motivators and Community Health Workers know the community. We could learn a lot from each other if we talked to each other more often, and we would achieve more by working hand-in-hand to reach the common goal of good health and a better quality of life for the people.

It would help if the people working in the hospital knew more about what the Care Groups do. For instance, if all the nursing students were to visit the Care Groups during their training in Community Health, they would discover that the Health Team and the Care Groups are both important and that they need each other.

We Care Group Motivators, and others who work in the community, like the CHWs, also sometimes share the blame when community health planning is not as good as it could be. We are often scared to speak out for our community, because we are employed by the Health Service and we fear for our jobs. This is a pity, because a grass-roots worker who is always with the community knows the people and understands their joys, problems and worries, and can be the voice of the community. It would be very helpful in the planning of community projects if supervisors would assure their grass-roots health workers that nothing will happen to them if they tell the truth about the community's feelings.

Another problem is that our seniors who are working in the hospital often lack confidence in the people's abilities. It would be good if they would visit the groups more often to see what is happening in the communities, and what Care Group members can do. People from the villages can do many things if we teach them correctly and give them a chance, but in many areas where supervisors do not know the communities they do not allow real decision-making at the grass-roots level, and only lip-service is paid to community participation. It is only when both sides know each other that the community members will gain more confidence and become empowered to work together with the Health Services, and the Health Services will have enough confidence in the community members to allow them to share in the decision-making process.

A career structure for community workers

The Care Group Motivators have gained strength. They are able to start projects on their own, without my help. They are slowly losing their fear of contributing in discussions with their superiors and can talk freely to them, which they did not dare to do before. However, the formal qualifications of Care Group Motivators are still those of nursing assistants, and the Motivators remain at this level in the Health Service structure, however much additional training and experience they have.

One of our greatest handicaps as Motivators has always been that our loyalties are divided. We are caught between the demands of the hospital management and those from the community. We have two masters: the hospital and the Care Group Top Executive. The fear of losing their jobs affects the way people work. Mostly, when Care Group Motivators do not do things properly it is because of the fear that, if they do not do the things the way they are told, they are going to be fired.

Even with all my experience, I am also afraid. The only reason why I can talk freely to the doctors working with us in the Care Group Project is that I am very much used to them. But before I would talk the same way to any other person in a higher position, I would first look very carefully at what type of person he is. There is a Tsonga proverb, 'Do not wash your feet in the spring before you leave the place, because tomorrow you will want to drink from it.'

I hope that one day there will be a proper career structure for Care Group Motivators, so that they will not simply remain in the lowest position in the Health Service hierarchy for all their working lives. Promotion could be based on length of service and on gaining additional skills and experience. Maybe, in the future, people who want to work in the community will no longer have to start by training as assistant nurses or CHWs, but will be able to train as Motivators by doing courses in community development or other topics that will be useful for work in the Care Group Project.

5. A dream: working together for better health

If I close my eyes I can see a wonderful picture of how we might work together to reach the goal of adequate Primary Health Care for all:

At the beginning of the year the hospital Health Team and the Care Group Motivators sit together and plan the work in the community for the year. Then the Motivators bring the plans to the Care Groups, so that the members can look at them and decide what contributions they can make – for example, supporting a vaccination campaign. Because the groups know about such activities well in advance, they can fit them into their yearly plan. The Health Service organisers also tell the Motivators about any problems they have noticed in the area, and the Motivators talk to the people in the communities to find out what they think and what solutions they suggest.

When it is time for the vaccination campaign, the hospital Health Team and the Care Groups work hand in hand. To start with, six weeks before the campaign is due to take place, the Motivators revise the subject with the Care Groups, and talk about the campaign at the meetings. The Care Group members decide how to inform the community and organise the campaign. Each Care Group makes its own plans, quite independently. The activities are quite different from community to community. Some groups arrange meetings and others act plays. Some make songs about the disease, and others arrange for somebody to come and talk about it.

When the health team comes to do the vaccination they find a community that has already been informed about what is going to happen. People know about the disease to be prevented, and its dangers. The Care Group members have planned how to support the health team, and allocated group members to the different places where the team will be working, to help with organising the people. The campaign is very easy, and everybody is happy.

Many benefits result from working more closely together. The Community Health Team and the Care Group members have had a chance to get to know each other, to learn to respect each other, and to hear about each others' problems. After seeing how well the Care Group members were communicating with the health team, the people in the community trust and respect the Care Group even more.

The Motivators and their supervisors also really listen to each others' views. And after seeing what the Care Groups can do, the supervisors no longer find it difficult to allow decision-making to take place at the grass-roots level. The Care Groups now have a real chance to become important actors in the task of promoting health in their communities as partners of the public health team.

We are not working for health alone, but for everything that concerns the well-being of the community. All the people working in community development meet regularly to discuss what each is doing, and give each other ideas. From there, we go on and see what can be done together, make plans, and act on them. It can no longer happen that the Agriculture Department is doing development projects, and the Care Groups are doing health, and the two are totally separated. Everybody realises that you cannot have health without food, and you cannot provide food unless you are healthy and can work.

Now the dream is beginning to come true

That was my dream five years ago, when we talked about the story of the Care Groups up to the 1990s. In the year 2002 it has still not all come true, but – as we describe in the next chapter – a lot of things we hoped for are beginning to happen. Above all, the group members are becoming more mature and independent, and we have a new Co-ordinator who is bridging the gap between the hospital services and the Care Groups. Also the work of the Care Groups is being appreciated more and more by the Government Health Services, which are at last involving the Motivators in community programmes and activities.

Chapter 9

Care Groups in the New Millennium

La tivisaka hi ye xaka

The real friend is the one who informs you without hiding anything

Chapter 9

Care Groups in the New Millennium

The previous chapters in this book are based on interviews in the 1990s. This chapter, based on recent reports and conversations with Selina, brings the story of the Care Groups up to date. In the last few years, a lot has happened – and some of the hopes that Selina expressed in the last chapter have begun to be fulfilled.

An important event in 2000 was the opening of the new Matimu Training Centre at Valdezia near Elim. A new Co-ordinator, Buyisile Mdhlovu, has been appointed. She is a nurse with a lot of experience in AIDS education, and is co-ordinating the Care Groups' HIV/AIDS programme. Selina, who has been Acting Co-ordinator, is introducing her to the work in the Care Groups – and at the same time learning from her about HIV/AIDS prevention.

The new Co-ordinator has already helped the project to make progress. One of her many achievements is that as a trained nurse she has been instrumental in closing the gap between the Care Groups and the nurses in the hospital. Now there is good co-operation between the two.

Another important change is that there is increasing public recognition of what the Care Groups have accomplished, and a new appreciation of what well-trained volunteers are able to do. With the new emphasis on Community Based Health Care, administrators have come to realise that in places where Care Groups have been working for some years there is already a solid basis on which to build. The Government Health Services appreciate the work of the Care Groups in the fight against HIV/AIDS, and have invited Care Group Motivators to participate in workshops for training trainers. Because the Care Groups are well known, it is easier for them to gain people's confidence and talk about matters that were previously taboo.

The expansion of their work is very encouraging for the Care Groups, but has also brought new challenges. There are not enough trained Motivators to go and start groups in every community. New methods

Once a Care Group has been started, two members come to us for training on one subject that the group feels is an urgent problem. Nowadays, this training is often on HIV/AIDS. Then they go back and discuss the topic with their Care Group, and the Motivators check that they are doing it correctly. Later, another two people can come to be trained on another topic. That way, each group will have its own experts on various subjects, and can function on its own.

2. Care Groups and HIV/AIDS

Only a few years ago, Selina was concerned about whether it would ever be possible to overcome the very strong taboo against discussing sex. As in many other countries, there has been a remarkable change since HIV/AIDS became a matter of public concern.

Taboos about discussing sex are breaking down

It was when I was in Kenya in 1995 that my eyes were opened about the problem of AIDS. It was the first time I saw people suffering from this disease. At that time people did not believe what they were told in health education. They were convinced AIDS was caused by evil spirits which take the flesh and leave skin and bones behind.

It used to be very difficult to talk about sex, but since HIV came it has become possible. Care Group members can now talk with other women about sex. It has even become possible for me, although I am a woman, to talk to men about it – and in the fight against HIV/AIDS it is very important to work with the men as well.

You can only talk with people about things that are normally taboo in our culture when they trust you. This happens when you are known because of the other work you have done. For example, early in 2000, I organised workshops for headmen in a new area, to teach them about chlorinating the water because there was a danger of cholera after the floods. Later, because they knew me, they helped me to organise workshops where we discussed HIV/AIDS and breast-feeding. It was because they trusted me that I was able to talk with them about these things.

Talking about sex used to be difficult

This extract from an interview with Selina in 1998, about the problem of sex education, shows how rapidly the taboo against discussing sex has broken down in the last few years.

One thing which should be included in a health worker's training is sex education, especially when there is the new problem of AIDS. However, I am not sure how far Community Health Workers or Care Group members will actually be able to help families on this issue, or on others, like illegal abortion. In Western culture it is the parents' duty to tell the children. In our culture, somebody else has to tell. It is not yet well accepted to talk to your own child. I do try to talk to my own daughters about family planning, but even we can't talk freely about it. They just say, 'We know'.

In a way, it is a good thing to have initiation schools when the girls reach maturity. In South Africa, circumcision of girls is unknown. This is important, because circumcision of girls is a terrible thing. With us, girls' initiation schools are purely educational, to introduce them into adult life as women. It is the traditional way of telling them what they should know.

A nurse at one of the clinics once did something which surprised us. She saw that all the girls were going to initiation school, so she also went. It would be a good thing if more nurses would go to these schools. They could influence the teaching of the girls and make sure the information they get is reliable. But this applies only to initiation schools for girls. A nurse should not go to boys' initiation schools, which are dangerous and where the boys are still circumcised.

Health Services should come up with a good idea about sex education, but they must do this together with the community. The final solution should come from the people. Here the two cultures could meet.

Now, when we have workshops for headmen and chiefs they are very flexible and free, and they are fighting against the taboos about not talking about sex. They ask interesting questions. I have sometimes been surprised that they came from the men, for example, 'What happens when a woman continues breast feeding when she is pregnant?' (This was taboo before, and not allowed.)

The Care Groups and HIV/AIDS education

Today, all the Care Group members have been taught about HIV and AIDS. They must know that HIV is a virus, and that AIDS is when a person infected by HIV gets the different diseases that follow. In many areas, we have started a more intensive training programme, and we are extending it into other areas. To begin with, two members of each group attend a 3-day workshop. At the end they get a certificate.

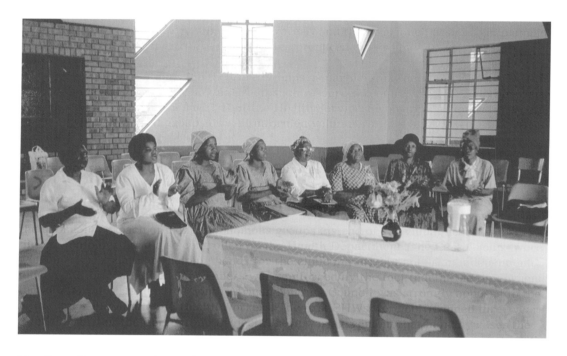

The Care Groups now have their own Training Centre. The picture shows members attending a course on HIV/AIDS. (Photo: M. Morier-Genoud)

Since the chiefs and headmen are so important in supporting the work on HIV/AIDS education, after the Care Group members have had their 3-day workshop, separate workshops are organised for the chiefs. They also get a certificate at the end. Then they organise a community meeting in their own place, where the two specially trained members of the local Care Group and the chief give HIV/AIDS training to the community. Not all the areas have been covered yet, but this work is continuing.

Recently, the chiefs were invited to Pietersburg to hear Nelson Mandela speak on the problem of AIDS. They said that we Motivators should go with them. When we got there, the people in charge of the meeting refused to let us in, as it was only for chiefs – but the chiefs protested, and said they must let us in because we were the people who had taught them. So we were able to hear the talk on HIV, which was very good. The chiefs were very interested. Ever since that meeting they have started asking a lot of questions, and they actively encourage their fellow-chiefs to go for HIV training.

The Care Groups are now planning to extend their educational activities to traditional healers and pastors. The church is important. They must know that praying is not enough. The churches are too slow, and have not done enough yet – some of them even continue to resist the use of condoms.

In our training sessions, we explain about HIV in a way the people can understand. We explain that a woman who has HIV can pass the virus to the child during birth, and she can also pass the virus on to the child through breast-feeding. When Care Group members do house visits they inform everyone about breast-feeding and AIDS. When we train the Care Groups we also invite the elderly for training. When the old attend the workshop it will encourage the young, because the older people are the heads of the extended families.

Advising mothers

After a woman has delivered a baby, the nurse tells her that if she has any problems she can contact one of the specially trained Care Group members, whose names are pinned up at all the clinics. This helps people to gain confidence. Recently Elim hospital got a special award for 'Baby-friendly Care', because a Care Group next to the hospital goes to the waiting mothers and the maternity ward in the hospital, and to the market place, to talk about how HIV can be transmitted from mother to child, and about breast-feeding and AIDS. Their health education is easier to understand than that given by many nurses because the Care Group members talk like the people talk, rather than giving formal lectures.

Recently, the hospital at last began to give treatment to HIV-positive mothers. But they only get the treatment if they have already been for a test and are known to be positive. This is one reason why we tell people how important it is to go for testing, which is now free of charge for everybody. Unfortunately, there are still mothers who did not go for tests and have not been treated. For them, we have to consider most carefully what advice we should give about breast-feeding.

Very poor people already do not breast-feed enough, because they have no time while working on the farms to earn money. Then the child has no resistance. Because not every child from an HIV-positive mother gets AIDS, at present we advise the mothers that the best thing to do is to breast-feed exclusively for the first 3-4 months, not giving the baby any other food. (Food other than breast milk – either the porridge traditionally given to very young babies, or powdered milk – can cause diarrhoea if utensils are not clean, and the use of powdered milk leads to malnutrition if the mother cannot afford to use enough.) With this short period of breast-feeding the child does not get too big a viral load, and it gets through the first months with good nutrition and does not die from causes other than HIV. After that we recommend the mothers to stop breast-feeding and give the child maize-peanut porridge.

The fact that many mothers cannot afford alternatives to breast-feeding is just one of the things that shows how much AIDS is related to poverty. HIV is a virus that can infect both rich and poor people, but they will not react the same. The rich person has had good food and is healthier and has more resistance. Rich people are better informed and know how to protect themselves. If they are sick, they can go to a doctor, and they have medical insurance. Rich mothers who are HIV-positive can feed their babies with powdered milk, which poor people cannot afford. Indeed, a poor woman may be forced into prostitution to feed the family. I personally know of a woman who earned a living by sewing, and when the sewing machine got broken she had no money to repair it. So her only way out was to sell her body.

Living with AIDS: counselling and support

Reducing fear and stigma
The more you know the better you are protected. If you are negative you must do everything you can to avoid getting infected. If you are informed, you can live more healthily, use condoms, and eat better. What we have to do is to live positively, to give a hand to

those who have AIDS and to help those who are sick. Before the Government introduced testing for everybody, we encouraged people to join the Treatment Action Campaign (TAC).

Now that tests are available, Care Groups are encouraging people to go for blood tests when they feel they might have AIDS, or have lost a lot of weight – and if they are positive, to tell someone. Before, they did not tell and did not go for tests, because they were afraid they would lose their jobs. That did often happen. Now there is a new law in South Africa that employers are not allowed to dismiss somebody because of HIV/AIDS, but unfortunately not all keep to the law.

Recently the Care Groups have started a Counselling Centre where people who have any kind of health problem can go for advice and information – for example mothers of malnourished children, or people who want to know more about HIV and AIDS, or have been diagnosed as HIV-positive and want advice. People can stay at the Centre for several days until they feel that they can cope with life at home.

It is very important to do everything for all, not exclusively for people with HIV/AIDS. This helps to avoid people being stigmatised, and being afraid to go for help. The same is true for home visits. Motivators and Care Group members visit everywhere, not only homes where there are AIDS patients. If people are sick or old or disabled and cannot cook for themselves any more, and there is nobody to look after them, Care Group members cook for them, and they get vegetables from the Care Group community gardens. This is something Care Groups do for all old, sick and disabled people, not only those with AIDS.

Counselling and support for AIDS patients and their families

People who have been diagnosed as HIV-positive are especially in need of counselling. They are worried and often despair when they are suddenly faced with the prospect of becoming ill and dying. At the Centre they are encouraged to live positively despite the disease. They come to realise that if they give in, they will die, but when the process has been explained to them, and they understand how to fight it with good food and a positive outlook, they will live longer. The same is true for the ones who have actually become sick. People who just stay under the blanket, not leaving the room and avoiding all contact – or even being rejected by their own people - will die very soon. If they receive counselling, explaining how they can still live positively, they will discover that they are loved. This is very important.

Towards the end of 2002, our Co-ordinator helped AIDS patients to start a support group where those affected can exchange their experience and discuss their problems. This does not involve Care Group members because the topic is too sensitive. Already, many more such groups have been formed in some places. Now some people with HIV infection can stand up and say openly that they are positive. This will help to break down fear.

Care Group members are doing a great deal to support patients and their families. With the training we have given them, they are able to tell people how to care for AIDS patients in the family, and to know what is infective and what is not. Care Group members are helping the patients' families not to reject them, but to accept people with AIDS in their homes, and to cook for them, wash them and look after them.

The Care Group members also support the relatives who are struggling to cope with the situation, and try to help them to achieve a peaceful atmosphere in their homes, and avoid quarrels. This also helps the patients. Finally, they prepare the patients to

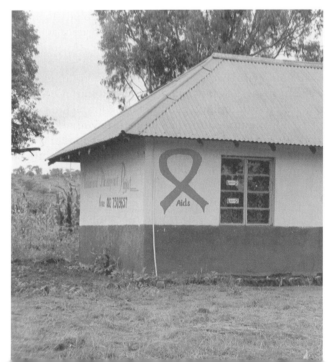

A village house where young people can come to get information on HIV/AIDS (Photo: M. Morier-Genoud).

be content to die at home, and talk to the family so they are also less scared of death. When a patient dies, the Care Group members go to the home, and people accept that death. The Care Groups also care for children who have become orphans because of AIDS or for other reasons. They look after them until the Social Worker has arranged a permanent solution for them – and also make sure that they do not feel too lonely and miserable at times when families get together, for example by arranging a Christmas party for them.

Helping with TB treatment

As there are many people with HIV/AIDS who also have tuberculosis, some Care Group members asked for training in TB so they could help with their treatment. The aim is now to train all the Care Group members. When patients are discharged from the hospital they are often still very weak and almost unable to walk. The trained Care Group members go to the patients' homes and give them their tablets. They stay with them, chatting with them, until they are sure that the tablets have been swallowed. They can tell by listening to the way a patient talks whether he has swallowed the tablets, or is keeping them under his tongue, to be spat out as soon as the visitor has left. Care Group members do not allow this trick! As soon as the patients begin to recover and are able to walk, the Care Group member encourages them to start taking exercise, and they have to go to her home to get their treatment.

This shows me that the Care Groups have really grown up! Many years ago, as I mentioned in Chapter 6, the doctor in charge of the TB ward thought Care Groups could be useful to supervise the treatment of the patients at home *(the DOTS 'direct observation' strategy, recommended by WHO)*. At that time it was not yet possible. It would have been too big a responsibility, especially as the doctor wanted the project to start almost at once, and there would be no time for proper training. Also, there were many taboos about TB which made patients shy to talk about it. Now the Care Group members themselves asked to learn about supervising the treatment, because the time was ripe for it.

Health education for men

Four years ago, a male Care Group Motivator at one of the other hospitals started to invite the men to meetings, because he found it important that men should also get health education in general, and be taught about HIV/AIDS. At that time it was still difficult to talk about AIDS. He held yearly meetings, inviting doctors from Johannesburg to speak at them. Every year more men attended – this year there were 1200! Now he will try to form smaller groups, which could work like Care Groups.

We hope that this education will eventually reach the traditional healers, because they give a lot of wrong information. They tell men they must have sex with a child or a baby to protect themselves from AIDS, or to get rid of it if they are infected. This is one of the most horrible results of the fear of AIDS, and is resulting in more and more babies and young girls being violated. Important men and doctors may be able to convince the men that you cannot cure AIDS by ill-treating children. The best way is to protect yourself from catching the virus by using a condom.

Partners in the fight against HIV/AIDS

The Government is now doing a lot. It is involving the Care Groups in its efforts and has adopted the Care Group idea of using unpaid volunteers. The Care Group Motivators have been invited to workshops organised by the Government to train trainers for HIV/ AIDS work.

There are many new organisations dealing with HIV/AIDS, such as youth groups and women's groups from certain churches, and we try to work hand-in-hand with them. However, some have a rather different way of working. For example, some organisations pay their volunteers, which causes confusion – but so far the Care Groups have never asked for money. They are still strong, and we Motivators support them and give them courage.

Some of the volunteers are young people with very little experience, and they only do the work they have been told to do. I have nothing against young people, but it is best if their efforts are directed towards work where they can be especially useful. It is very important to involve young people in HIV/AIDS work, because when they take part in campaigns and in running youth workshops the young people will follow them.

However, there are some things the Care Group members can do better than younger people or people from outside the community. Because they are mature and experienced women, when they visit a patient's home they can look around and see what they can do to help. And because the Care Groups have been around for such a long time, and people trust them, they can tackle sensitive issues like HIV/AIDS and TB, where outsiders – who are often met with mistrust – would fail.

The sad thing is that all these activities to fight HIV and AIDS are too late. The Apartheid Government kept quiet and did not talk about it, and the new Government was too slow to do something. I do not think any particular person is to blame that it took so long. At the time the epidemic started there were too many other big problems in South Africa.

3. Men and Women

Men and Care Groups

In the days when most of the men went away to work they were very surprised when they came home to find a newly-built round house and a toilet, fruit trees planted in the yard, a clean family and a well-dressed wife who was attending the Care Groups and was a garden member, and was happy working together with the other women. Some of the men became jealous and ill-treated their wives, but many were very happy with their wives. Some Care Group members said that their husbands told them never to stop attending Care Groups, because they saw that it was a good thing. They were proud of their wives.

However, there are very few men who are members of Care Groups themselves. Most of the groups are women only. There are many reasons for this. One is that traditionally, men and women don't discuss topics like children or venereal diseases in mixed groups.

We originally thought that today, when many men have come back home because they have lost their jobs, they would be happy to join some activities like the Care Groups. But this is difficult.

Husbands who are jobless and back from Johannesburg feel very bad and start drinking and do not care for the family. This means that the mothers have less time to be at home, because they must go out to look for work. They leave the children at home, and the children do not get enough food. In any case, the money the mothers earn is not enough to feed the family. A man feels very shy when he is at home and the woman goes out to work, and she becomes the breadwinner. He feels the woman is now looking down upon him, and he thinks he is losing his qualities.

When we try to motivate the men to join a project, they do not like to do something for no money. They often do not believe that women work voluntarily in the Care Group – they think that the women are employing and paying each other. Men want to earn with their work. They want a job. This is why it is difficult to organise the men into starting a project. With women it is easier. We wanted the men to start a workshop to produce solar cookers for the community. I discussed the idea with one man, and he looked at the solar cooker to see if he could do something. He tried to get other men to join, but at present there is nobody who is interested in starting such a thing.

Some years ago, in one community something very interesting happened. A group of men did decide that they wanted to join the local Care Group. They told the Care Group members that they were going to join the group. But the women said, 'No, we don't want you to join. You have never been interested to do work without being paid. Why are you coming now? And if you join our group, you only want to be the ones who direct everything. If you want to join the Project, you'd better start your own group.' So the men started their group, and discussed what they could do. One of the men said that he was suffering from the mosquitoes at night, because there were always water pools in the *donga* (a gully caused by soil erosion) near his house. So the men worked on the *donga* to remove the pools. They also started a community garden. This Care Group still exists, but now there are also many women who have joined. It seems that men alone can't manage, so they asked women to help. Men cannot do it without somebody supporting them.

Women are now empowered

Many families stand because the women are strong. When the Project started, many men were away from home because they were contract labourers and had their jobs in town or on a farm. The women remained at home with the children. It was easy for the men to forget about their families and remarry in town. The women made plans to work as a group and to support each other, in order that the children would have food to eat and could attend school. Women now do many things that were previously men's business. For example, they build houses themselves, or are improving their houses. The women now have more responsibilities.

Since the change of Government, in the New South Africa, people have become even more independent. They don't want to be told what to do any longer. The women ask many questions and want to know exactly why we want them to do a certain thing. They want to decide for themselves whether a particular action should be taken or not. It is now more difficult for health or development professionals to use the community for carrying out something an organisation wants to have done, because people want to organise themselves. I am happy that now that the people feel free to say anything or ask anything, or explain their position.

This is real development towards self-reliance, and it makes me very happy. But it is still an important issue for us to inform the women about their new rights and help them to stand up for them. For example, there are still many women in rural areas who think that men have the right to beat women. They don't know that in the New South Africa the law is now equal for all, men and women, Black and White.

4. A final summing-up

There are a few things I would like to say at the end of this last chapter, as they are the most important lessons I learnt during the 28 years of working with the community. One does not need to be educated to improve the environment around oneself. I did have the opportunity to attend training courses, but I still say that Care Groups are my University, because I learned most from the people themselves.

I have learned that community development projects which people initiate themselves are sustainable, because they feel that their own needs are addressed. People at grass-roots level are able to improve their standard of living if they are given a chance to do so.

Facilitators who are helping the community with a project should consider the customs and values of the people in that community. If they respect the people, even if they are different or strange, they will also be respected and accepted in their turn. For example when the people eat with their fingers, the facilitator must do the same when offered food.

When communities are striving to meet a certain objective they also gain self-reliance and human dignity, and this is permanent. This encourages them to continue to help themselves. Community development is a learning process. Each step that people take to reach a certain objective makes them able to do the next step better, which will improve the next project they undertake.

Full participation of the community is important. People should not only be asked to contribute when their labour is needed, but be allowed to take part in all the steps of project management: thinking, decision-making, implementation and evaluation. When this happens, development projects strengthen the community. The people are able to organise themselves and their leadership will be strong. Once the community has learnt to solve a particular problem this leads to further development, as they will be keen to find ways to solve other problems, and it will be easier for them to do so.

In my heart I feel very happy. All the time during my work I used all my strength and knowledge so that what I intended to do should be successful. Now I am happy that the community can do it themselves, and that the Care Group Project is in good hands, and the good work will continue even after I have retired.

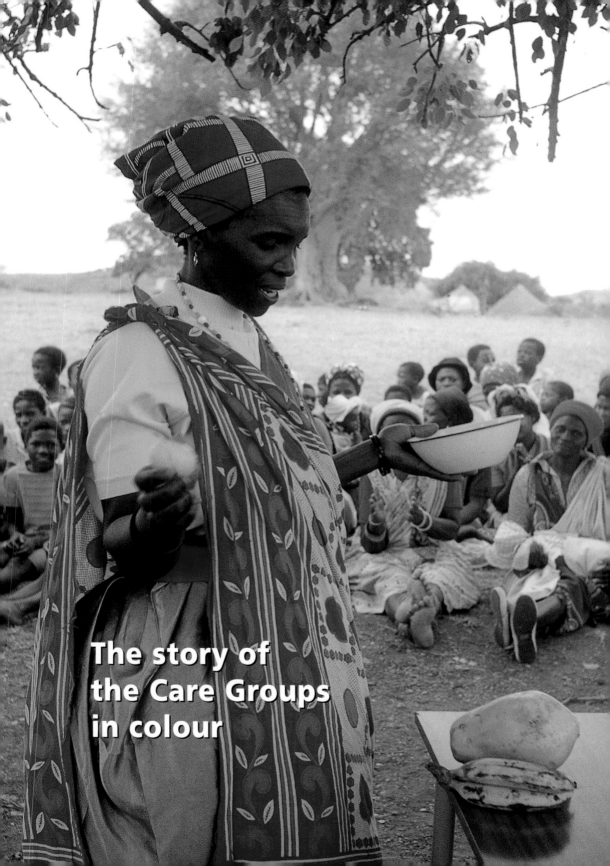

The story of
the Care Groups
in colour

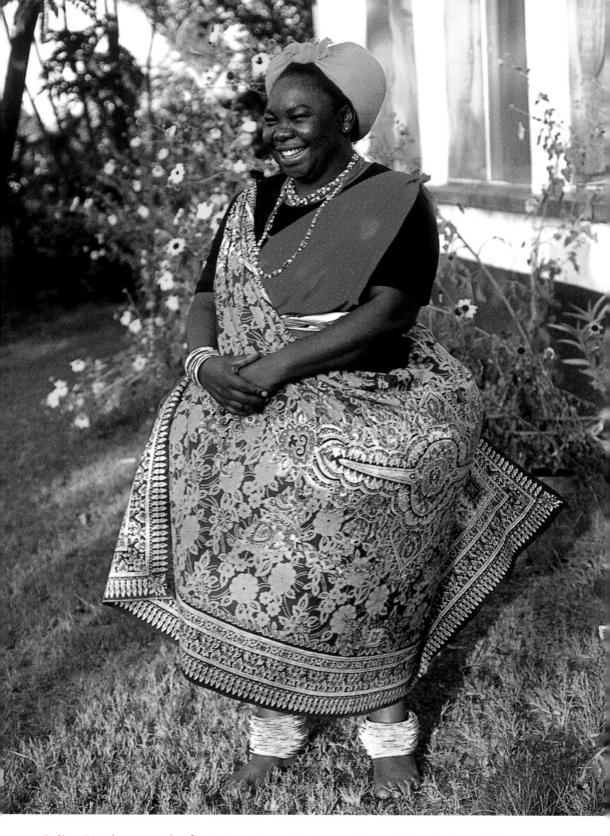

Selina Maphorogo, the first Care Group Motivator, in traditional dress. (Photo: E. Sutter)

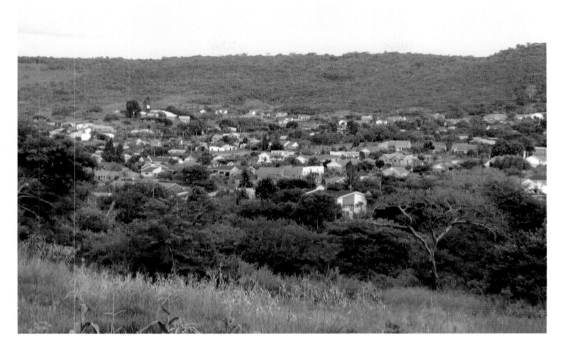

Selina's location. (Photo: M. Morier-Genoud)

A recent picture (2002) of Selina Maphorogo in the "Educational Tree Nursery" by her house. One purpose of the nursery is to demonstrate how to cultivate seedlings for tree-planting projects. (Photo: S. Horber)

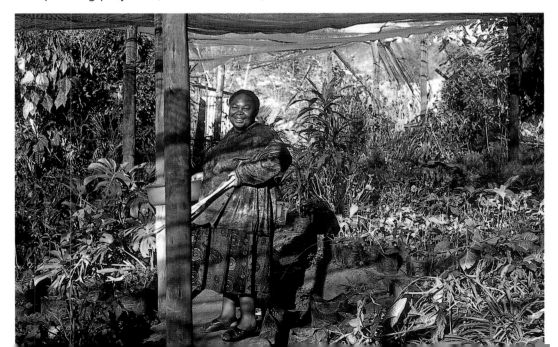

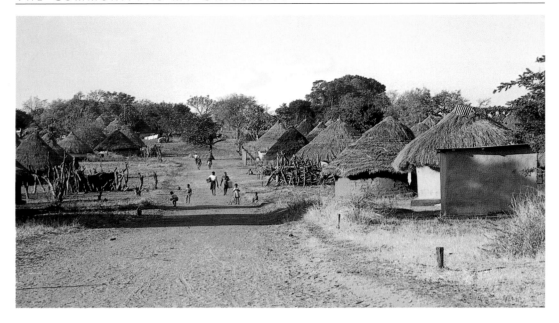

Setting the scene; one of the many villages near Elim where the Care Groups work. (Photo: E. Sutter)

Selina visiting a village home. From the old ladies, she learned many things on which she could build in her work with the Care Groups. (Photo: E. Sutter)

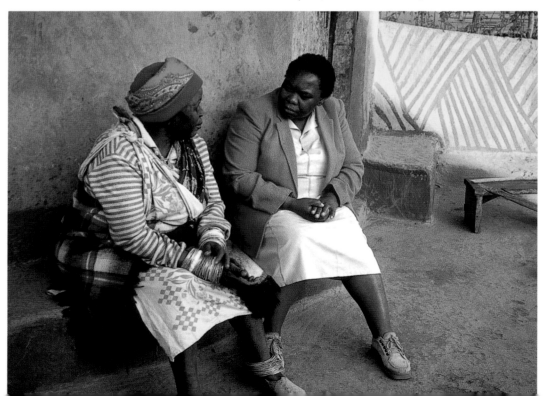

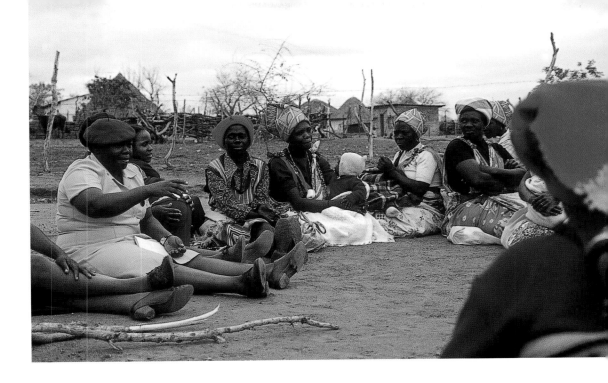

Above, a Care Group meeting. 'A good leader does not sit high up on a chair. She sits on the ground where the group members sit'. (Photo: E. Sutter). Below, Care Group members learning to examine eyes for trachoma. They practised on each other before visiting village families. (Photo: E. Sutter)

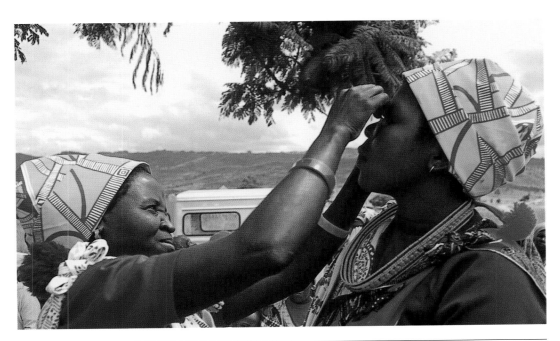

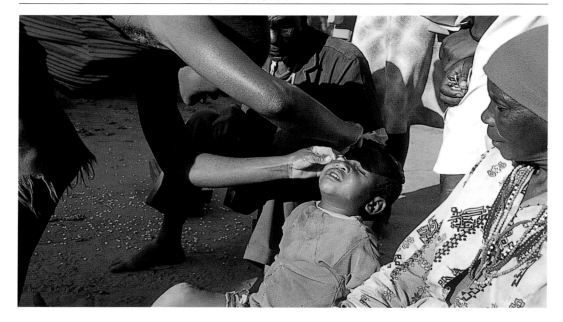

Visiting a family and examining a child's eyes for trachoma. One of the Care Group members is keeping a record in her notebook (see illustration, p. 100).
(Photo: E. Sutter)

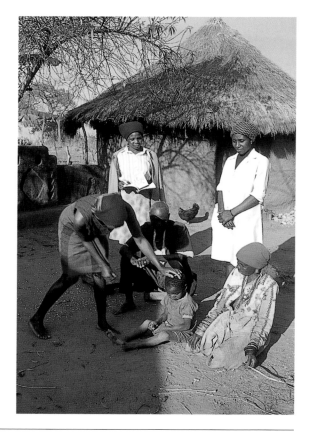

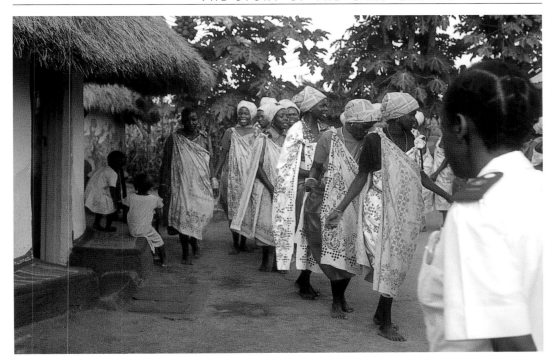

The Care Groups soon developed their own way of working: 'First the whole group went dancing and singing through the streets ... The people came flocking, and then the group told them what they had learnt from the Motivators.' (Photo: E. Sutter)

Care Groups have many ways of introducing new ideas about health. In this picture members are presenting a message about nutrition at a local festival. (Photo: M.- A. Gneist)

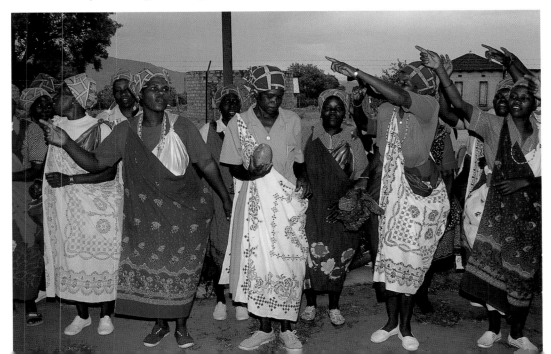

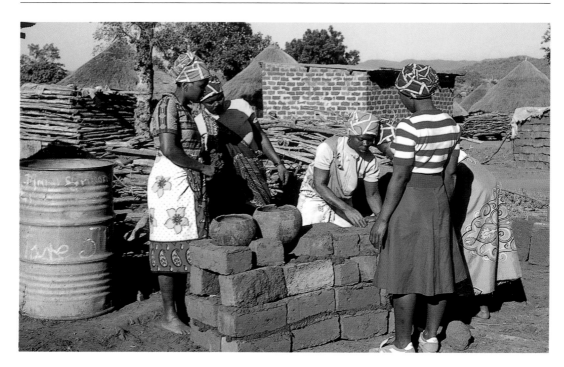

When trachoma had been largely brought under control the groups looked for new activities. They started on projects like building mud stoves to save fuel, and gardening to produce fresh vegetables. Communal gardens are one way of involving poorer members of the community. The lower picture shows a garden with a mud stove where Care Group members are demonstrating how to cook vegetables. (Photos: E. Sutter)

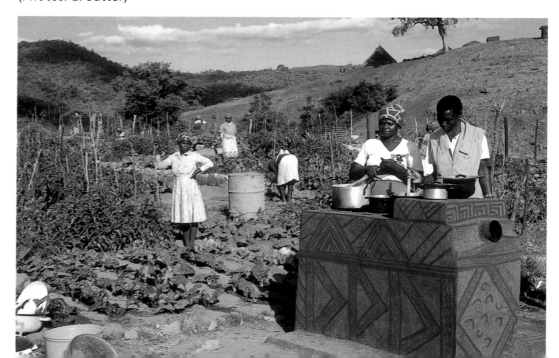

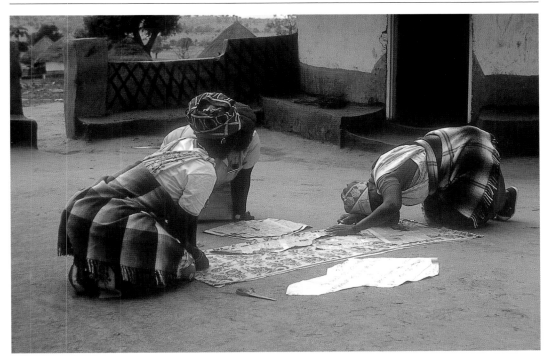

A group making 'wonder boxes'. This is another way of saving fuel (see pattern in Appendix, p.266). (Photos: C. IJsselmuiden)

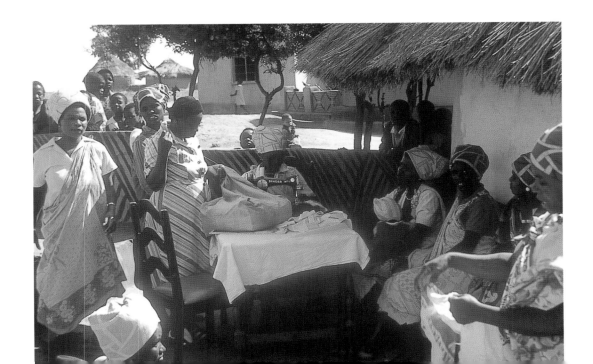

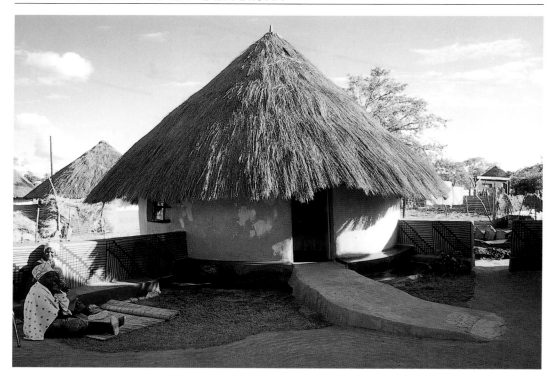

Care Groups are helping the disabled and the elderly people in the villages. Above, a house where a ramp has been built to allow wheelchair access (Photo: S. Horber). Below, a discussion with a group of elderly people about organising activities (Photo: E. Sutter).

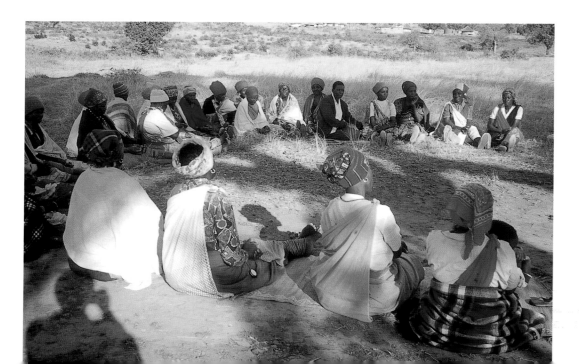

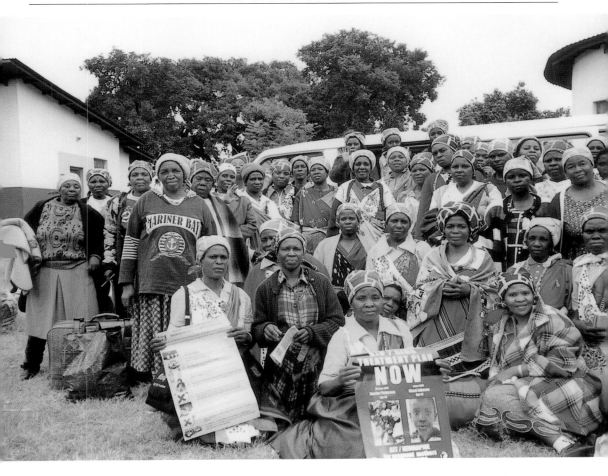

The Care Groups respond to new needs as they arise. This picture shows members attending a workshop on HIV/AIDS. They are at the Care Groups' new Matimu Training Centre. (Photo: M. Morier-Genoud)

'The Care Groups are still strong after 25 years because they taught us a lot of things that are improving our lives and homes ... We also share what we learn with our neighbours and with neighbouring communities.'

Statement by a Care Group member (page 98)

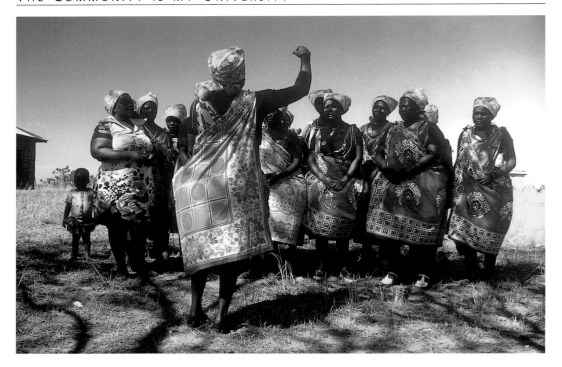

(Photo: E. Sutter)

The Care Groups are still full of enthusiasm after nearly 30 years – as this Care Group song demonstrates:

A Care Group Song

Whatever happens I will stay with them till I die (2x)
This, this, this community,
This, this, this Care Group,
With the Care Group

We ourselves are happy with the Care Group (2x)
With the Care Group (3x)

Speaker:
We build mud stoves
We plough the gardens

Chorus:
Whatever happens I will stay with them until I die.
etc.

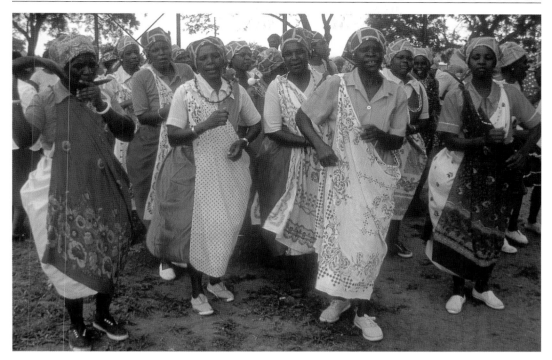

(Photo: M.- A. Gneist)

Risimu ra care gurupu

Hambi swi nga va ka njhani ndzi ta fa na yona (2x)
Leyi, leyi, leyi community,
Leyi, leyi, leyi care gurupu,
Ka care gurupu

Hi ta tiphina ka care gurupu (2x)
Ka care gurupu (3x)

Speaker:
Hi akana switofu
Hi rima na swirapa.

Chorus:
Hambi swi nga va ka njhani ndzi ta fa na yona.
etc.

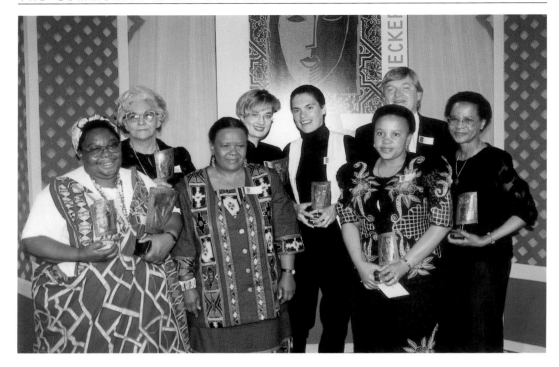

In 1996 Selina Maphorogo received the South African *Woman of the Year* award.
'At last my country recognised the value of the Care Groups' (On the extreme right is
Dr. Mamphela Ramphele with the award for education). (Photo: Checkers-Shoprite)

The same year, the Care Groups celebrated their 20th anniversary.
(Photo: C. IJsselmuiden)

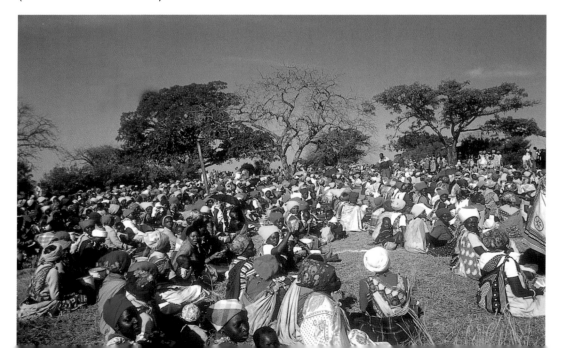

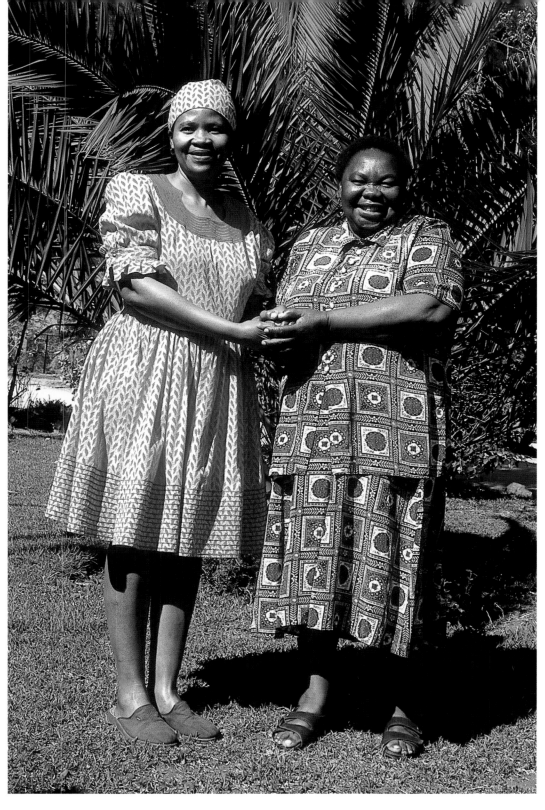

A new phase in the history of the Care Groups begins. Selina Maphorogo handing over to the new Care Group Co-ordinator, Buyisile Mdhlovu. (Photo: S. Horber)

Postscript:
From health problems to an understanding of health and well-being

Erika Sutter, Carel IJsselmuiden and *Peter Kok*

Some of the reflections in this chapter concern issues that the authors were not aware of when they were busy with the day-to-day work of the Care Group Project. They are insights that are the result of looking back over a quarter of a century of the project's development. All the people involved might do some things differently if they could start again. Nevertheless, they are convinced that the Elim Care Groups offer an effective model for health care that is truly based in the community.

2. The achievements of the Care Group movement

The first achievement of the Care Groups was a dramatic reduction in the prevalence of trachoma in the area. This surpassed all expectations – in the first 2-3 years after the groups started work, the prevalence of intense inflammatory trachoma decreased by almost 50%. The prevalence decreased even in places where the disease was not actively treated, because hygienic conditions improved rapidly in the villages where the groups were active. For example, people were encouraged to use individual face cloths, and to dig refuse pits to reduce the number of flies. Unlike the treatment of individuals, these community activities benefited everyone. Even though after 3-4 years most groups had stopped focussing on trachoma control, the prevalence of the disease continued to decrease until in the mid-1980s it practically disappeared (Ballard et al. 1978, Sutter & Ballard 1978, 1983).

Decrease in the prevalence of intense inflammatory trachoma (TI) and entropion in relation to the duration of Care Group activities, 1976 – 1995

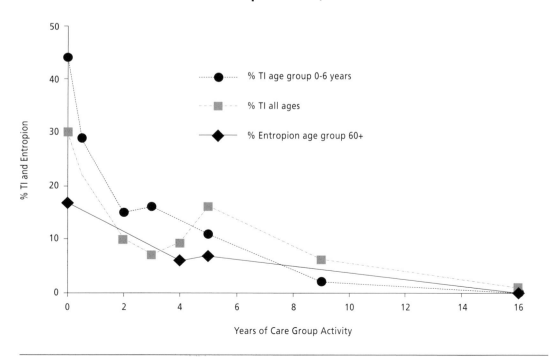

The blinding complications of trachoma, trichiasis and entropion, which take many years to develop, also became rare. During the first years of the project, 200 or more cases of entropion annually were treated surgically at Elim hospital. By the time the project had been active for about 10 years there were only 5 - 6 cases per year, and the number has remained at this low level ever since. Unfortunately, resources were not available to carry out an extensive study comparing the prevalence of trachoma in areas with and without Care Groups. However, the higher standard of environmental and personal hygiene, and the general high level of health consciousness in the population in the area where the Care Groups are working, have certainly contributed a great deal to the sustained control of the disease (Sutter & Maphorogo, 1996, 2001).

Once trachoma was being brought under control, the groups turned their attention to a broader range of activities in health promotion and development. The results of many of these are clearly visible. A communal vegetable garden can be found in every village where there is a Care Group. There are settlements where each household has built a mud stove to save fuel and reduce the risk of childhood burns. Some groups have built crèches for the children of working mothers, and others have built toilets, or modified the houses of disabled people so that they can move in and out unaided in their wheel chairs. We cannot present numbers demonstrating an improvement in child health, because this was not systematically surveyed from the beginning, due to the lack of resources for monitoring and evaluation that exists in most routine health service settings. But experienced Motivators and nurses at the clinics have observed an improvement in the nutritional status of the under-fives. Many people have learned how to prepare a high-protein and high-energy weaning porridge with maize and peanuts. Many have also learned about Oral Rehydration Therapy (ORT), and know how to prepare the rehydration fluid themselves from sugar and salt, so they are not dependent on getting ready-made mixtures from commercial or other sources.

The improvements in the homes of Care Group members did not only enhance the quality of life of their own families, but also had a 'ripple effect' in the whole community when neighbours observed the changes and began to introduce these themselves. Because the Care Groups have always emphasised the need to address problems of poverty and underdevelopment as community problems that need community solutions, rather than as individual problems requiring individual solutions, the activities of the groups have improved the situation of whole communities.

The most important achievements of the Care Groups, however, cannot be pinned down in hard facts and figures. The Care Group members have developed an understanding of health problems, and have devised many effective methods of health education in the community. They have been able to take the lead in their villages in introducing new practices like the disinfection of water to prevent cholera, and building improved VIP toilets. Most recently, they have been concerned with educational work to increase awareness and understanding of HIV infection and AIDS. These achievements have now been recognised by the Regional Ministry of Health, which is now actively encouraging the founding of more groups – more than 25 years after the first Care Groups were started.

The groups have also had an important influence on the personal development of the women involved. Training in problem-solving and decision-making when addressing their own needs has strengthened the women's self-reliance and self-esteem, both as individuals and collectively. Even in the days of apartheid, when men and women were not equal in the sight of the law, the women in the Care Groups were learning to express their opinions and to speak out in public. When Health Committees were formed in the villages, often the only women who became members were from the Care Groups.

From the start the Care Groups have been flexible enough to adapt to the needs of the day, whether these were particular health hazards, natural catastrophes like droughts or floods, political unrest at the end of the Apartheid regime, or the challenges of the New South Africa. They have won the respect of the members of their communities, including the men, and they can fight for women's rights in a male-dominated society. They can even break old taboos – for example, as part of their AIDS prevention work they talk publicly about sex. Men are starting to listen when Care Group members stand up to voice their opinions. Many of the Care Groups have become a trusted force, and a useful platform for development in their communities.

As the movement has grown, its organisation has inevitably become more complex. Ongoing training in 'group building' finally led the groups to establish their own Care Group Council and Management Committee. They have become more and more independent of the base hospitals. The strength of the organisation was tested during a prolonged period when there was a vacuum in the Project's central administration. In spite of this, the groups continued to organise themselves, growing in strength and determined to pursue their own objectives. It was during this period that the members of the Top Executive were asked, 'What would you do if the Hospital Superintendent said the Motivators must go back to the wards and stop working for the Care Groups?' The answer was, 'We would go on, whatever happens at the top' (Sutter & IJsselmuiden, 1998).

3. Reflections on the development of the Care Group movement

Translating visions and plans into a community process

The earlier chapters of this book describe the translation of an idea into a thriving community project. It was a real stroke of good fortune for the Care Group Project that Selina Maphorogo was part of the team almost from the beginning, and has provided continuity by working as a key person in the movement until today. Her strength lay in the fact that despite her intimate contact with a western type of life style, and her training as an assistant nurse in the hospital, she did not reject her own culture as being inferior, and something belonging to the past, as many educated people tend to do. She remained deeply rooted in her own society, which she continued to love and appreciate. This enabled her to liase successfully between western 'scientific' cause-and-effect thinking and the more relational thinking of the village people. She found the words of traditional wisdom, the context and the ideas which could be incorporated in the thought patterns of the women of her community. Her special skills in communication, her compassion and respect for people, especially the poor and the handicapped, and her great patience in making sure that none of the members were left behind, were all essential in mobilising the women.

One of the cornerstones of health education and community involvement is the communication of western-style health messages in such a way that people can relate them to their own cultural concepts. Selina describes how she struggled to find her own personal solutions to the problem of bridging the gap between the two systems of thought. For her, the sharing of knowledge is a basic requirement at all levels of interaction, and it should always be a two-way movement, between expert professionals and the inputs from the community. Throughout the book, there are examples of this process. The key elements can be summarised as follows:

- Listen to the people and learn from them before you start to teach.

- Respect the people and their culture and adapt your messages accordingly.

- Allow enough time for people to ask questions, to discuss the problem, and finally to come forward with their own solutions.

The Care Group Motivators

Choosing the 'right' people to interact with the communities, especially in the initial phase, is crucial for the success or failure of a new initiative. Class differences, the stability of the staff and the leadership, cultural sensitivity, and adequate and ongoing training and support are all key issues that must be considered by anybody who wants to start something like the Care Group Project. Each needs to be specifically addressed in relation to local circumstances.

As the Care Group Project grew, more Motivators were appointed, and after a while they became responsible for all the day-to-day work with the groups. Nurses and other experts were co-opted for special occasions when expert knowledge was required. Selina and her colleagues were sensitive and innovative people, who could bridge the gap between the community and the Project Director and the hospital. Almost all of them were women who had had a minimal amount of formal school education, and had been trained as assistant nurses. The work was also supported at times by Community Health Workers (CHWs), who had a similar training and status.

The decision to appoint assistant nurses as Motivators was made because the Project Directors realised that they could interact more readily with the people in the community than most trained nurses could. For ordinary people in the community, the professional status of doctors and nurses meant that they were regarded from a distance, and approached with awe and respect. This attitude was reinforced by a culture that dictates that younger people, or those lower in the local hierarchy, should not speak after an older or more respected person has spoken. We saw how deeply embedded this attitude was during refresher courses for Care Group Motivators and Community Health Workers. If senior nurses were present, the 'lower-level' staff only felt free to talk after the nurses had left.

Even when they belong to the local culture, highly-trained professionals very often find it difficult to consider poor people as true partners in their work. This applies to nurses as well as to doctors. The average nurse comes from a 'better' social class, in which girls are more likely to attend secondary school. Once they are qualified, nurses belong to a closed profession with a strong tendency towards ever more professionalism. Hence both their family background and their professional training tend to remove them from the community from which they came. They are tempted to preach over the people's heads, without first listening to what they know already. Like expatriate experts, they think they know everything better anyway.

Nursing assistants, and others with a similar educational background and status, have fewer barriers to overcome in communicating with rural people. In socio-economic as well as educational terms they are almost on a par with the village community. In an atmosphere of mutual trust, people feel free to share their everyday worries with them. This sharing leads to a partnership in the struggle for a better quality of life. Messages coming from people whose life situation is not much better than that of the people with whom they work are likely to be more credible and more easily accepted by the community. The women appreciate having women Motivators to talk to, whereas the men prefer male counterparts.

Strengths and limitations of the Motivators

In retrospect, however, the question must be asked whether the decision to work mainly with the Motivators was a good one in terms of long-term planning. How much can one expect a local woman who is hardly literate, and has rarely been further than 30 km away from home, to achieve in terms of development and innovation?

Health workers in the community must be close to the people – but they also need to be respected as group leaders. This can only happen if they have a well-founded knowledge of the message they want to pass on. Without this, they cannot translate medical jargon into the people's own language, nor can they engage people in discussions based on their own experience and traditions and lead them to reach their own conclusions and follow this with appropriate action.

The Motivators were very successful in carrying out this process of translation in the early days of the Care Group Project. Trachoma was a disease that was already known in the community and was perceived as a problem. The Motivators had both a sound knowledge of the disease, and a good reputation as friends of the people. This enabled them to encourage the women to join a Care Group to work for a common aim, with a clear plan of action, and to propagate the idea over a wide area.

It was when the prevalence of trachoma in the area had been reduced, and the interests of the groups shifted to other fields of health and development, that the limitations of the Motivators became apparent. They themselves felt overtaxed, and were afraid that they would not be able to respond adequately to the groups' demands. New inputs from outside were required to keep up the momentum of the Project. This is especially important in rural communities, where there is a static population not exposed to the rapidly changing 'outside' world. New ideas were provided by the Project Directors, who explained them to the Motivators, who then had to pass them on to the groups. This was the speediest way to act, but it proved to be the least effective. It often failed, because the Motivators lacked personal experience of seeing such new ideas put into practice, for example by projects elsewhere. They felt very unsure when carrying out the instructions we had given them. In Selina's words, 'When you are just told what to do you get nervous, because you are afraid of not doing it correctly.'

A process of 'translation' was needed here, too – to translate the ideas of the Project Directors into terms the Motivators could understand and pass on. It was also necessary to encourage the Motivators to express their own views about the proposals that were made. One way in which the 'power gap' between the Project Director and the Motivators was reduced was by adopting a simple rule in Project meetings: although new issues could be raised at any meeting, and everyone could speak to them, no decision could be made within 2 weeks of an issue being raised for the first time. While this sounds like a recipe for delay, the opposite was probably true; the delay in decision-making allowed the Motivators to discuss the matter among themselves, and return with a shared decision a week or two later. Once this decision was taken, it would hold and be implemented. So rushing would actually have been counter-productive.

Limitations of 'grass-roots' health workers as agents for change

Many community-based health projects have depended on workers who came from the community, and whose cultural background, socio-economic status and educational level were similar to those of the people with whom they worked. They have been given a variety of names at different times and in different places: 'Village Health Workers', 'Barefoot Doctors', 'Community Health Workers', or 'Motivators'. To avoid confusion, in the following discussion we use 'grass-roots health workers' as a general term.

Grass-roots health workers were expected to be advocates for the people of their community, and to bridge the gap between them and the health services. They were supposed not only to attend to the health needs of the individual, but also to be agents of change. They were expected to promote measures such as environmental sanitation, and link with workers in other sectors such as agriculture and development, so that they could all work hand in hand, responding to the community's needs.

In practice, grass-roots workers have often been successful in providing some care for individuals, but they have generally not been able to fulfil the hopes vested in them as agents of development and change. This is hardly surprising, since the tasks they were expected to carry out were often beyond the capacity of almost any individual, and certainly outside the scope of a person with a minimum of formal education, often working alone. This has led to much debate in the last decades about whether health workers coming directly from the community are useful at all.

The other expectation was that grass-roots health workers would bridge the gap between the community and the health services. This has also proved to be very difficult. One reason is that in many places they have been employed and paid by the Health Services, even though the original concept was that such workers would be chosen and supported by their own communities. As Health Service employees, they have tended to identify more with their employers than with the community they were supposed to represent.

The experience of the Care Group Project throws some light on the strengths and weaknesses of grass-roots health workers, and on ways in which they can be helped to fulfil the expectation that they will provide the impetus for development. The Motivators were mostly local women whose lives had been spent in the same area. They had been to primary school and then gone to Elim and other local hospitals for training as assistant nurses. Their strengths in communicating with the village people and working in partnership with them were evident from the beginning of the Project. However, they did also have their limitations, and because we (the Project Directors) failed to recognise the true nature of these, we devoted little thought to how best to assist them in their progress.

Unfortunately, it was only after we had left the Care Group Project that we identified the following three main factors which may have limited the ability of many of our Motivators to act as agents for development. We have no doubt that these factors could be effectively addressed, but we have not had any opportunities to find ways of doing this in practice. The limiting factors we identified were: firstly, the restricted horizon of a person with little formal education who has hardly ever travelled beyond the immediate community; secondly, a culturally-determined lack of long-term vision for people who have little sense of the future; and finally, the difficulty poor people have in 'owning their own mistakes', and evaluating what they have done with a view to moving forward. Below, we discuss some of these problems and suggest solutions to them – or at least, things we might have done differently.

A restricted horizon

Grass-roots health workers, who have generally grown up and found jobs in the place where they were born, have neither the financial means nor any inclination to travel around merely for the sake of opening their minds for personal enrichment. A journey to town to visit a relative in distress is often already a major undertaking.

Having staff members who are content to stay in one place does, of course, bring benefits to a project. They bring continuity in personal relationships and in the project's objectives. However, the disadvantage can be stagnation and a lack of new ideas. It is only exceptional people like Selina who, through untiring efforts, manage to widen their horizons, but nevertheless continue to be rooted in the local culture and do not move away to work elsewhere. These are the people who become agents of change.

Many grass-roots workers lack personal contact with people or projects in other areas, and have neither seen nor heard about how people elsewhere solve their problems. Learning by reading books is not really an alternative for people whose culture depends much more on oral tradition than on the printed word. They are not accustomed to reading books for their own interest or pleasure, and it is a difficult undertaking for people whose level of literacy is hardly sufficient for rudimentary daily needs, especially if the books they are given are in a language in which they are not very proficient. With hindsight, we can see that it would have been a good idea to develop strategies from the beginning to increase the exposure of the workers in the Project to ideas from elsewhere, through training, travel, video, visits, or other means.

Concepts of time and planning for the future

The request for 'more time' has been a recurrent plea in Selina's story. 'Time' was a constant source of friction between us, the Project Directors, and the Motivators. We all happened to be Europeans, but we think the problem would have existed even with African directors, since their professional training and different experience would have separated them from the traditional society. As Selina commented, 'In town it is different!'

The problem was not only that the Motivators and the people in the community needed time to absorb ideas, and to go at their own pace when they started putting them into practice. This we could understand, though we found it hard to learn the necessary patience. Something we found harder to understand was why we had so many difficulties when we tried to train the Motivators in planning future activities. There seemed to be barriers against actually implementing the theoretical knowledge about planning, and against recognising planning as a basic requirement for the operation of any project.

We had to acknowledge that long-term planning was not an attribute of people rooted in this particular traditional society, but although we were conscious that the problems arose from deep-rooted cultural differences, none of us could define their nature at the time. After returning to Europe, we learned more about the meaning of time in African traditional societies. One cannot generalise, of course, and African cultures – like any others – change with time and with the intensity of outside contacts. One African scholar pointed out that the concepts of pre-colonial Africans have been undergoing changes ever since the first contacts with Europeans, and the changes have become more rapid with the impact of neo-colonialism and globalisation. Today, people in Africa live with both European and traditional concepts of time. The clock is important for programming activities, but for existential matters traditional concepts prevail (Dr Josef Kalamba, personal communication).

There are African cultures, like that of the Akan peoples in Ghana, where the future plays a very important role (Gyekye, 1995). But there are others where the future is not an important concept. For example John Mbiti, writing about Kenya, says:

'… time is simply a composition of events which have occurred, those which are taking place and those which are immediately to occur.(…) Traditionally time is two-dimensional with a long past, a present and virtually no future. The linear concept of time in western thought, with an indefinite past, present and infinite future is practically foreign to African thinking. (…) Partly because of western-type education, together with the invasion of modern technology, African people are discovering the future dimension of time. (…) But the change from the structure built around the traditional concept of time to one which should accommodate this new discovery of the future dimension is not smooth.' (Mbiti, 1969)

A similar comment is made in a more recent book by Boon (1996), who is writing about the Khosa, Zulu and Sotho peoples of South Africa, whose culture is close to that of the people in the Elim area. He says that 'Westerners accept that there is an internal locus of control, and that, to a considerable degree, one can determine one's future', whereas the African 'accepts that there is an "external locus of control"', and that, 'There are forces operating in every person's life over which he or she has little or no control.'

These analyses helped us afterwards to understand the reactions of the Motivators when we wanted them to make plans for the future. But at the time we simply found it frustrating. Conflicting concepts of time should be an important theme in training workshops. Although Western health and development organisers and their African colleagues may know in theory that different cultures have different concepts of time, in practice, they still find it difficult to understand each others' attitudes. If all the people involved in a project become more aware of what is at the root of the problem, this may lead to better mutual understanding, and a balance may be found for fruitful common planning and implementation of activities. To quote John Mbiti again: 'Both sides need to reach out to each other. The African will need to take seriously the crucial importance of the future in an undertaking that is intended to become sustainable, and the Westerner will need to try and accept the essential importance of the past to the African.'

The difficulty of 'owning one's failures'
In refresher courses for Motivators or for Care Group members, we often included evaluation exercises. The aim was to look at the successes and at the failures, in order to learn from them. But we felt that this was the least-appreciated part of the programme. The sparkle of learning something useful and new was missing, and we noticed a certain resistance to doing the exercises we suggested. Why did we have to repeat again and again that it was most important to evaluate what had been done? And why was it so difficult actually to do it? Mamphela Ramphele, herself a South African, indicates one possible reason:

'One needs self-confidence and self-esteem to be able to acknowledge one's failures and weaknesses. The humiliations of conquest, racism and poverty have undermined many people's self-esteem by labelling them as mistakes of God's creation. How can we expect them to own mistakes?' (Ramphele, 1995)

Training, career structures and hierarchies

Training
Selina Maphorogo has stressed the importance of training many times in this book. She herself had to learn 'on the job', and though she was successful in the end, she suffered a great deal from doubt and uncertainty while she was working out for herself what she should do. She feels very strongly that health workers should not be sent unprepared into the community, but first be appropriately trained. When they start working, they need support in the difficult task of initiating a community process. Even when they have more experience, there should be an adequate support structure for them – they feel too

often that they are left on their own in the community, where they have to take difficult decisions unaided.

In the Care Group movement, there was an all-time low point after some years of activity, when the Motivators reached a stage where they had nothing new to give to the groups. They resorted to repeating old topics, and many members left. It was clearly urgent to increase efforts to train the Motivators. Weekly in-service training sessions did not help much, because most of the time was taken up with discussing urgent logistical problems encountered during the preceding week, and this left little space for new inputs. Annual refresher courses did allow ample time for in-depth discussion of the topics covered, but once the Motivators were back in the daily routine of group meetings they needed more encouragement than we could give them to apply what they had learned. We realised that theoretical training courses did not help much, because their school education had never taught them to transform theory into practice.

Various other attempts were made to upgrade in-service training. We tried producing a periodical containing teaching material, but it was not actually read by those for whom it was intended. People who are barely literate are not in the habit of reading unless it is essential. Some Motivators did attend courses run by other projects, like the Valley Trust, and passed their new knowledge on to the groups. But unfortunately, most of them were either too shy to venture into the unknown, or they were simply not proficient enough in English.

The decision we finally made was to give Selina the opportunity to go to England for a course in community development and adult education in the University of Manchester. She was already playing a most important role in the Care Group movement, and she had always been willing and able to seize every possible chance to go to training courses or visit other projects and learn new skills to pass on to the groups. We considered that if she had more formal education she would be able to plan and carry out appropriate training courses for the Motivators, and the whole movement would benefit.

However, when she had completed her course and returned to Elim, ready to become the trainer for the Care Group Motivators, Selina encountered a number of barriers. Her fellow-Motivators found it hard to accept that her knowledge was now superior to theirs – a common problem for anyone who has grown out of a fellowship of 'equals' and has acquired new qualities. In addition, there was resentment because she had been singled out by the expatriates, in particular the 'Eye Doctor'. Not only had she been given special treatment, but she had been enabled to attend a University course without having the paper qualifications usually required. In a hierarchy-conscious society, this was a further cause of friction.

The situation gradually resolved itself, and the Care Groups have recently opened a Training Centre of their own. Nevertheless, it is clear in retrospect that there is a danger that promoting one person may do more harm than good – even though that person has special gifts. If we could start again we would ensure that all of the people working in the project were offered opportunities for personal advancement. Some would doubtlessly respond more enthusiastically than others, but they should all have a chance. People who did not respond at all could be channelled back to duties for which they were better suited than for work in a development project.

Personal advancement for the Motivators could include opportunities to see other ideas and practices at first hand. It should be possible to set up an extensive networking programme where project staff would be exchanged between various health and development projects in their own country, and even abroad. These exchanges could be coupled with training in community development and adult education. However, such a programme would require more funds and more time than most donor agencies would be prepared to allocate to development projects. Donors want to see a project progressing fast, without long delays for training staff.

Career structures and hierarchies

Although some Care Group activities are financed by NGOs, most of the Motivators are still employees of the Health Department. However, they remain officially in the grade of assistant nurse. Within the present structures, there is no way of recognising the fact that the capabilities of experienced Motivators have grown far beyond those of their counterparts in the hospital setting. They have worked for years in a job with a lot of independence and responsibility, and had a lot of additional formal and informal training. The problem of establishing a career structure that takes this added competence into account can only be solved at the level of the Health Department or the Nursing Council – and at the time of writing it has not yet happened.

Having a proper career structure for the staff of a project is most important if a project is to be sustainable. If there is no chance of making progress in their profession, there is a danger that the best people may leave and go elsewhere, so that it will be difficult to find leaders who have an inside knowledge of the project. Another danger is that staff members who remain may not be interested in learning anything new, since without the prospect of a better salary there is little incentive to spend extra energy on one's personal upliftment.

The Care Group Project was fortunate in that Selina and the majority of her colleagues never gave up improving their knowledge and skills, in spite of the low salaries and the fact that the additional training brought no prospect of advancement in the nursing hierarchy. This enabled the Project to survive and grow despite various changes in the leadership. After 12 years of expatriate Project Directors, a highly-qualified local Co-ordinator took over the administration of the Project, and was active in initiating new structures – the Care Groups Association with its Council and Top Executive, which provided a framework in which members of the Care Groups in the communities could participate in and support the Project leadership. The existence of this new structure benefited the Project greatly when, in 1993, all the highly qualified senior staff left for personal professional advancement, and Selina had to step in and take over the co-ordination, unprepared for that particular job. It was only recently, shortly before her retirement, that she was able to hand over to the new Co-ordinator, a South African nurse.

Relationships with the hospital's administrative structure

At the beginning, the Care Group Project was simply the Eye Department's outreach programme, busy with trachoma control. The ophthalmic nursing staff felt they were part of the new venture because the Project had been conceived and realised together with them, and they supported it. To this day, the staff of the Eye Department at Elim Hospital see the Care Groups as their 'own' project, and practical sessions with them are still part of the curriculum for ophthalmic nursing students.

As long as the community work remained a specialised eye care project, the senior nursing staff in other departments of the hospital had no reason to become involved. The situation changed when the Care Groups turned to general health promotion, and even more when they moved beyond health and engaged in village development and income-generating activities. The Motivators were no longer simple health workers, but also development agents. By trial and error, they had gradually become experts in fields that the nursing management staff, not trained in community development, knew little or nothing about. This resulted in a very difficult situation. The senior staff felt threatened by having subordinates whose duties they themselves did not really understand, and the Motivators felt that they were misunderstood by their seniors and colleagues within the hospital.

In retrospect, we have to ask ourselves whether the situation would have been better if we had involved the hospital's nursing administration from the start in the planning and implementation of the Care Group Project. Inexperienced as we were when we ventured for the first time into the community, we had simply not realised that the 'Doctor / Nursing Establishment / Care Group Motivator' relationship could ever pose a problem. We did not realise that it was possible for a structure to stand in the way of a good concept. It would have needed more energy and time to involve the senior nurses of the general hospital as well as those of the eye department in our planning. In addition, in the beginning the Project was a trial with a highly uncertain outcome, so we preferred simply to get started, and worry about the administrative red tape later.

The Care Group Project is by no means unique in having by-passed the hospital hierarchy. There are many development schemes that have been initiated by doctors, who are often more free to operate than nurses, and have more power to persuade policy-makers to support community interventions. The doctors often tend to ignore the nursing staff of their institution, partly because they find it difficult to deal with the rigid hierarchical system in the nursing profession. The nurses, in their turn, feel that they are not taken seriously. They are rarely involved in the planning stages of a project – even when, once it has started, they will have to supervise the Primary Health Care workers.

In a book on Community Health Workers, Gill Walt (1990) stresses that when a new health scheme is started, all sections of the institution in question should be involved in some way in the planning and implementation. There are examples where this practice worked to the benefit of all involved, for example the Manguzi Village Health Workers' Project in Kwazulu/Natal. Selina suggests in Chapter 8 that when plans are made to establish Care Groups in new places, several members of the hospital team in the new area, and not just the future Care Group Motivators, should visit existing groups to find out how they function. We shall never know whether we could have given our Project a better start if we had tried to involve the whole of the hospital administration from the beginning. There might have been less antagonism, and we might have found more common ground. On the other hand, in the South African context, where the hospital Matron was bound by the restrictive rules of the Nursing Council, the planning process might have become so frustrating that the Project would never have got off the ground at all.

In recent years, the situation has changed for the better. One reason is that the Government Health Services are beginning to value the work done by the Care Groups, and co-operate with them. Another change is that with the appointment of a new Co-ordinator who is a qualified and experienced nurse, relationships with the nursing hierarchy have substantially improved.

4. Establishing Community Based Health Care: the Care Group experience

Community Based Health Care (CBHC)

The term 'Community Based Health Care' (CBHC) stands for health-promoting activities at community level, provided by the communities themselves, on their own terms. CBHC is the most important and basic element of an integrated and comprehensive health care system in which all actors, from the community members to the referral hospital, will play a responsible role. The work of the Care Groups fits very well into this definition of CBHC, although when the Project started nobody would have described their activities by this name.

The experience of the Elim Care Groups showed that there are a number of necessary preconditions for the successful implementation of CBHC. One reason for the success of the Care Groups was that many of these conditions were fulfilled, or if they were not, local solutions could be found. These enabling preconditions are discussed in detail in the next section. They include a political environment that allows for change, and an enabling health system. It is important to have a common concern that is shared by a large section of the community, and a response to it that is acceptable and understood. There must be people able to bridge the gap between the ways of thinking of the 'health professionals' and the members of the community. Finally, there must be enough time for the process to take place.

Enabling preconditions for implementing CBHC

A political environment allowing for change
A positive political environment is an important contributing factor to the success of organised CBHC. In the best case, the local political power is willing to allow and even support a movement for change, and is prepared to take the risk that change may challenge the traditional order of society, and even alter the distribution of power relationships determined by gender, money or other factors. It is also important to have a system in which reallocation of resources is not impossible, so that staffing and finances can be rearranged in the light of new priorities.

It frequently happens that those in power are unwilling to take the risk of allowing community action that may lead to change. However, in a situation where the political background is one of violence, the members of a community may see interdependence as the only chance of survival, and this may make people willing to engage in common life-saving activities even when this means doing things which might not have been culturally acceptable under more normal conditions. The Care Group Project is remarkable in that it was a women's movement that started in a situation where women were marginalised for three reasons: they were women, they were Black, and they were living in former Gazankulu, one of the most neglected rural areas of South Africa. According to both apartheid and tribal laws they were lifelong minors with no legal rights, and they were socio-economically isolated because most of the able-bodied males were working far away in the cities.

The growth of the Care Group Project is an example of people seeking strength through group action even when the political system was not exactly supportive. During most of the first 20 years of the Care Groups' existence, under Apartheid, the political authorities felt threatened by the growing empowerment of women. The secret Security Police tried to suppress the movement towards change that the groups were bringing about. However, thanks to the fact that the Care Groups were a non-political organisation, and thanks to the diplomatic way Selina and the group members approached the local village authorities, most Care Groups enjoyed local support and continued to function despite an unsympathetic government.

An enabling health system

A comprehensive health system which included Primary Health Care (PHC) had already been introduced in South Africa before the Care Groups started work. PHC was introduced cautiously, in a form which was not supposed to pose a threat to the Apartheid doctrine. In fact, 'comprehensive primary health care', with nurses as the primary caregivers, was developed for the 'Homelands' only: it would never have taken off in the affluent 'White' areas. Ironically, although Primary Health Care was intended as 'second-class care for second-class citizens', it was nevertheless an enabling factor for community involvement in health, since it did allow the Project Directors to ask successfully for staff and funds to be transferred from hospital-based care to community-based primary care.

A common community concern

It is widely accepted as a basic tenet of the implementation of CBHC that when a programme starts it should respond to the community's own concerns. In the area where the Care Groups were founded, the high rate of blindness due to trachoma was such a concern. The disease was not only a public health problem in the opinion of health professionals, but one that was also very visible to the people themselves. In retrospect, it is clear that trachoma control was an excellent entry point for our community work. The transmission of infection was easy to explain, without overwhelming the village women with a multitude of facts, and there were many popular beliefs and observations about the disease on which to build. In addition, the field of action was limited, and the women could actually see the results of their preventive measures and treatment within the first two years. Their success in virtually eradicating trachoma in their area gave them satisfaction, pride and self-confidence.

Although in the past public health programmes were often centred on a particular disease, nowadays it is generally considered that it is a better policy for interventions to be health-centred rather than disease-centred. However, the Care Group experience shows that in certain circumstances a disease-centred intervention may be a good way to start. Their success in addressing trachoma, which was a recognised problem in the community, and one that could be solved by community effort, made the Care Group members aware that their efforts could have a real impact. They also observed that measures for trachoma control, such as household hygiene and environmental sanitation, helped to prevent other common diseases of poverty as well. In Selina's words, 'When we tackle one problem we solve five others at the same time.' This strengthened the women's confidence in their ability to solve problems, and prepared them for new ventures in health promotion and village development. As a Care Group member put it, 'We started with eyes, but now we can prevent many diseases in our community.'

People able to bridge cultural gaps

Doctors and nurses trained in western traditions tend to assume that people will immediately begin to tackle a health problem effectively if they are provided with knowledge about cause and effect, for example through education or 'social marketing'. The Trachoma Team from Elim Hospital started in the same way. However, the model did not fit traditional thinking, and simply explaining cause and effect was wholly ineffective in communicating with the community. It was Selina Maphorogo's insight into both cultures – that of the village women and that of the health professionals – that enabled her to construct a bridge between the two systems of thought, and this made it possible for effective communication to take place and lead to action.

Enough time for the process to take place

Effective community action requires the transformation of a task to be done into a community process. This process of translation and incorporation of new ideas is often frustratingly slow for the people who initiate projects. To the 'outside' expert the new ideas seem to be of obvious importance for survival in a rapidly changing and threatening world. There are life-saving interventions which should not be delayed. As the Chilean poet Gabriela Mistral put it, 'The child's name is Today' (quoted in Morley & Lovel, 1986). There will always be a conflict between the speed of action that the Health Services or project leaders deem necessary and the slow pace of consciousness-raising and decision-making in the community. There is no easy way to change behaviour in a short time. However, when changes have been introduced in a right and culturally sensitive way, they are lasting and constructive. A community that has been convinced that change is important has a large potential for participation in concerted action.

We feel that the Care Group Project benefited greatly from the fact that mostly there was little or no pressure for rapid success. The people working for the Project at all levels, including its directors, were not dependent on it for the advancement of their personal careers, and did not have to keep up with timetables set by donors. There were times during the first years when the Project's leaders, and some outside critics, felt that progress was too slow, and that too much time was being spent on one disease-oriented intervention. But the groups taught them the lesson that in a community project it is worthwhile to go at the people's own speed, and do things as they themselves want to, so that they can fully 'own' their project without feeling they are working for someone else, either an individual or an institution. The fact that the project was allowed to grow at its own pace has been important for its sustainability. Too many projects fail because there is so much push to 'get things done' that the people for whom the project is intended are left behind.

Later, when donors did become directly involved, the issue of 'project time' as opposed to 'community time' was placed in the forefront of the negotiations. The absence of time pressure allowed projects to start slowly, to take enough time to build mutual trust, and to proceed at the pace the Care Groups and Motivators demanded and could keep up with. The Care Group members had time to organise themselves as coherent groups. The women could become conscious of their own involvement in community health, and mature steadily from passive, dependent receivers of services to self-reliant actors in health and development.

5. The Care Group Project: an NGO and part of the Government Health Services

Support for the Care Groups comes partly from the Government and partly from various non-governmental organisations (NGOs). This kind of public-private partnership project is likely to become more common as public resources for health care become more and more limited in many developing countries.

When the Care Group Project started, as an outreach programme of the Eye Department of Elim Hospital, it had no outside funding. The Hospital Superintendent supported community health activities, and was willing to allocate some of the hospital's budget (provided by the Government) to the Care Groups. Some staff members were shifted from clinical duties to work with the groups, and for a short period the hospital also provided tetracycline eye ointment for free distribution in communities. It was when the Care Groups started to diversify their activities, especially into areas like gardening and income-generating projects, that other sources of financing had to be found. This was the beginning of the mixed Government/NGO nature of the Care Group Project, which has remained a key characteristic of the way it has worked ever since.

Since the Care Groups had always worked closely with the Government Health Department whenever possible, when they diversified their activities beyond health they naturally invited other Government Departments, such as Agriculture, to become involved. This was a lengthy process, and at first the groups met with rejection. For the co-ordinators of the Project the new situation meant that in addition to dealing with the Health Department, they also had to argue with the Departments of Agriculture, Community Development, and Forestry. Government departments tend to have rigid structures which cannot easily accommodate new developments. For example, the Agricultural Extension Officers were at a loss when the Care Groups grew vegetables successfully with the 'deep trench method' which the women had learned from the Valley Trust. However, once the Head of the Department could be persuaded to go and see it for himself by visiting the Valley Trust, he was convinced of its efficiency.

From then on, the Project had the support of the Agriculture Department, and because the Care Groups are also officially part of the Health Department, this recognition resulted in the communication between the two Departments improving markedly. The Project was thus instrumental in generating interdepartmental communication and co-operation – something that would have been less likely to happen had the Care Group Project simply been an independent NGO.

Advantages and disadvantages of mixed support

Government support for Project staff
The Care Group Project has benefited in many ways from being part of the Public Health Services. The financial benefits were considerable, since most of the cost of salaries for Project staff was borne by the Government. In addition, the Project gained because the staff members did not have to use a lot of energy for fund-raising for the core activities, and could concentrate on their work. Continuity was guaranteed because the essential activities were not dependent on donors who might withdraw their support as their own interests shifted. When financial assistance was needed for a special project, the support from the Health Services also meant that donors were not difficult to find, since as salaries were not needed the proposed projects appeared to be 'cheap'.

The security that a government job provides for individual grass-roots health workers, who usually belong to the poorer section of their society, is another important argument in favour of partnership with the Health Services. In the Care Group Project, the fact that the staff appreciate having a government job has helped to ensure stability and continuity. Many staff members have stayed with the Project for more than 20 years. The fact that the Motivators are part of the pool of assistant nurses in their hospital also has the advantage that a Motivator who is not really suited to working in the community can go back to hospital work instead of losing her job. However, it can also mean that when a hospital is short of staff, Motivators can be withdrawn from the Care Groups and ordered to return to ward duties.

There are various disadvantages in having a mixture of public and private support. In any project involving co-operation between a number of organisations there will inevitably be tensions about priorities for action and allocation of resources. Every NGO has its own aims, which are determined by the vision of the donors who support it. These aims may not correspond with the policy of the government, which has its mandate as the representative of the people. This is something that was perhaps not considered sufficiently when everybody was busy with the day-to-day running of the Care Groups.

On a personal level, tensions can arise between staff employed by the government and those employed directly by the project. Ensuring a good relationship between these two groups demands much diplomatic negotiation, and this was another problem that was often neglected in the early days of the Care Groups, to the detriment of all parties.

The Motivators are often considerably harassed by serving several masters. As Health Service employees, they are answerable to the nursing administration. The senior nurses in the hospital, who are their immediate superiors, have never been personally involved in the Care Group Project and often do not understand what they are trying to do. In addition, the Motivators are responsible to the Project leadership – originally the Project Director, who was a medical doctor, and now the elected Top Executive. And finally, the Motivators are the people who are directly in contact with the local Care Groups and their communities, who also have expectations.

Political implications of Government support
In the days of the Apartheid regime, which regarded all development outside the Apartheid ideology with suspicion, it was a great help for the Care Groups that they had support from Government departments and were working within the government health system. A sympathetic Secretary of Health in the Gazankulu Department of Health and Welfare, and the support of the hospital's Medical Superintendent, provided sufficient leeway for the successful growth of the movement under an otherwise hostile regime. This good relationship protected the groups from threats of interference from the 'secret police'.

Though government support was valuable for the Project in those days, it also caused problems with acceptance. If a project is seen to be supported by a government, its image depends to some extent on the acceptability of that government. Though the Care Groups were a non-political organisation, as long as the Apartheid Government was in power their status as part of the official Health Services labelled them automatically as a creation of Apartheid. This was felt strongly abroad, and also within South Africa, where many of the doctors working in community health at the time mistrusted any organisation that had links with the Government. Locally, the groups were often confused with the Gazankulu Women's Association, which was created by the Government as an agency for Apartheid propaganda. This even resulted in the groups becoming targets of abuse during the period of unrest just before the change of government in 1994.

Internationally, it may have been because of South Africa's reputation during the first decades of their existence that the 'Care Group model' never became as well known in the world at large as it should have been. The political situation also had an adverse effect on fund raising. Some potential donors were reluctant because of the close relationship with the regime, while others, especially multinational concerns, were frightened of getting involved with a potentially 'subversive' organisation which would not toe the Government line.

6. Care Groups implementing Community Based Health Care

Care Groups: effective partners of public health services

If groups like the Care Groups are accepted as partners, they have the potential to be strong allies of the government in the promotion of health. Apart from specific activities that they undertake, like building latrines or organising AIDS education, groups can have a more general influence in awakening health consciousness and a will to change things for the better. This was apparent in the area where the Care Groups worked. Through the influence of the Care Group members on their neighbourhood, relatives and friends, health messages spread rapidly within their communities and even beyond. Many observers have confirmed that new ideas are more readily accepted in communities where Care Groups are active than in other areas, and that it is much easier to implement health interventions where Care Groups have prepared the ground.

The value of organisations like the Care Groups as partners in Community Based Health Care is evident, but actually making use of such resources requires considerable flexibility on the part of the professional staff of the Health Services, who are not generally used to working with organised groups of well-informed volunteers.

The response of the Government Health Services to the Care Group Project

For many years the response of the Gazankulu Health Department to the Care Groups was an ambiguous one. At first, the authorities felt uneasy about, or even threatened by, the unusual approach of using autonomous groups instead of individual health workers directly employed and also controlled by the Health Department. The Care Groups were welcomed as a source of helping hands for the clinic nurses, but not as an independent movement for change. The uneasiness was reinforced by the fact that, at the time when the Care Groups started, the South African Nursing Council was strongly opposed to the introduction of Community Health Workers. The first CHWs were only trained three years after the start of the Care Group Project. There was agreement that in many cases the aims of Care Groups and those of the Health Services were similar, but in the Department's own words, 'The Health Services have their own hierarchy to use for the achievement of their own objectives which is not compatible with the self-directing nature of the groups.'

Later, once the Care Groups proved to be successful and became well-known, the Health Department was forced to become more flexible and accommodate this unconventional working force in its PHC programme to some extent. Indeed, the Department even attempted to take them over as its 'shop window'. Nevertheless, the Care Groups remained autonomous. With the growth and empowerment of the Care Groups, the Project became a force to be reckoned with, and members were elected to health advisory committees and later to civic committees in their villages.

In recent years the collaboration between the Care Groups and the Government Health Services has become even closer. For example, the Health Services, the Care Groups and the traditional village authorities are working together in the struggle to control HIV/AIDS.

Partnership in practice

In the early years of the Care Group Project, when it was directed by doctors who were also working at Elim Hospital, the groups were involved in many of the activities of the hospital's outreach programme. But later on they were often by-passed in the planning of interventions like vaccination campaigns, although they could have made a most valuable contribution by informing and organising the people. When the Health Services did make attempts to collaborate with the Care Groups they were not always successful. As Selina mentioned earlier, the groups resisted being 'used' as a cheap labour force to work for salaried personnel for some objective which was not one of their own concerns, or which they did not understand. Some officials who wanted to use the groups at short notice for specific community interventions were disappointed by the lack of an immediate positive response. Members of the Health Service staff, who had been brought up in its rigid hierarchical system, were sometimes too directive. In addition, they found it difficult to adapt to the Care Groups' expectations that the Health Services, in their turn, would respond to the group's needs and priorities.

Even with goodwill on both sides, activities involving partnership between professionals and voluntary groups do not always run smoothly. Health professionals and informal, self-directed groups often have different priorities. When a Care Group carries out an intervention it is not always completed in a way that would satisfy a professional perfectionist, and the work is apt to be interrupted by other activities important to the members and the rest of the community, like ploughing or harvesting, or caring for sons or daughters attending initiation schools. It is difficult to use the Care Groups for the implementation of a long-term health intervention, because they tend not to maintain a prolonged interest in a single topic. Their interests change in response to the community's immediate needs. Even if some Motivators want to continue longer with an intervention, they have no power to enforce compliance – this would be contrary to the Care Group philosophy. They can only exercise friendly persuasion, and this may not function with all members of the community. Social and educational barriers may prevent their being taken seriously by the better-educated or the 'better off'.

The Care Groups are most effective in acting on problems which affect the members personally, and which they can solve with means they find appropriate. They are not willing to work on activities they do not themselves see as being of first importance. Erika Sutter had to learn this lesson at a very early stage of the Project. As an ophthalmologist, she had originally planned to use the Care Groups to develop a 'perfect' community-based blindness prevention programme. After dealing with trachoma control they should have been instrumental in preventing xerophthalmia and ocular trauma; they could have informed the community about glaucoma and cataract, traced cases, and motivated people to go for treatment. She soon realised that the groups were not prepared to be used in this way. They had other priorities.

Professionals in the Health Services need to adapt to the fact that the people in the community see health as only one aspect of life – a life which cannot be subdivided into separate parts. They also have to realise that working with an autonomous group is different from working with an individual employee, and that existing groups have their own dynamics, and often a history of doing things in a particular way. They will not necessarily change their way of doing things immediately in response to an impetus from outside.

7. The special feature of the Elim Project: community groups promoting health

There have always been people engaged in Primary Health Care who belonged to their communities, but they have usually worked as individuals. There have also been many local groups, like church women's fellowships, who included some activities like health education in their programmes. The Care Groups, however, were something new in South Africa: organised groups of people from the community, working voluntarily with the main aim of promoting health. This is the most distinctive feature of the Care Group Project.

There are many advantages of work based on groups rather than on individuals. The members of a group support each other, and groups thus have more power to work for change than an individual can have. It is easier to mobilise people into action when there is an active group in the community than to do it through an individual community health worker or through workers from outside. In a group, as people share their experiences, they gain a broader insight into their community's assets and inadequacies than a single person can. The Care Group members have become aware that poverty and underdevelopment are problems more of the community than of the individual, and need to be addressed collectively. A group also provides continuity, because even with a changing membership most groups maintain a stable core.

However, there are some things a group cannot do as well as an individual health worker who has had a specialised training in preventive and promotive care, which may include monitoring chronic patients, and in some countries diagnosing and treating common diseases, and referring patients to another health facility when necessary. The ideal situation would be for communities to have both – groups like the Care Groups, and well-trained individual health workers – each doing the things they are best able to do, as summarised in the table on page 249, and also supporting each other. This could provide a great potential for health care that would be really rooted in the community. Trained health workers could share their specialised knowledge with the Care Group members in their meetings, and the Care Group could keep them in touch with what is going on in the whole community. One Care Group member, describing this ideal situation, said, 'We inform the Community Health Worker what is happening in each corner of the community. When we see a problem we cannot manage, she can go and see. That is where we need each other.'

Comparison of Care Groups and individual, trained Community Health Workers (based on experience in the South African setting)

Care Groups	Individual Community Health Workers
Operate as a group, which can offer mutual support.	Operate as individuals.
No systematic training, define topics themselves. There is a danger that they may forget what they do not practice for some time.	Trained according to a set syllabus to suit their jobs.
Respond enthusiastically and effectively to problems they have identified and to which they have found their own solutions.	Perform prescribed tasks as instructed by supervisor.
Work when they have time – and cannot be pushed!	Fixed working hours.
Focus on the community and the environment.	Focus on the individual.
Unpaid volunteers: - Cannot be ordered to perform specific tasks health management deems to be urgent. - Respond to emergencies slowly, because a task formulated by the Health Services needs to go through a community process. - Are unlikely to maintain a prolonged interest in a single topic; interests change according to their own priorities.	Payment in cash or in kind: - Tasks determined by health management. - Can respond quickly to emergencies. - Duration of an intervention is decided by the supervisor.
Empowerment enables group to work for change.	Less potential to become agents of change.

8. Care Groups in a global setting: other models of community participation in health

Community participation has always been an integral part of Primary Health Care as it was formulated in the Alma Ata Declaration. However, there are many ways of interpreting 'community participation'. An international group of health professionals who wrote about the topic during a course offered definitions that ranged from 'paying taxes so that the Government can provide the services' over practical activities, like building clinics or looking after relatives in hospital, to situations in which planning, priority-setting and the provision of services are done by a truly representative group of people from the local community. This last is what the Alma Ata Declaration intended, stating that Primary Health Care:

> 'requires and promotes maximum community and individual self-reliance and parti-cipation in the planning, organization, operation and control of primary health care, making fullest use of local, national and other available resources.' (WHO 1982)

Several authors who have examined the way in which this aim has actually been put into practice in health development in rural communities in poor countries have come to the conclusion that there are few successful examples of true community participation, in the sense of an organised structure in which the community has reached a measure of autonomy in planning and decision making, and control of the resource base. In most programmes participation has reached a level of 'co-operation' rather than participation, with a distant agent in control of the process and observing the expected outcome. (Chambers, 1983; Cohen & Uphoff, 1980; Hilton, 1998; Macdonald, 1994)

Many health programmes describe their activities as Community Based Health Care (CBHC), but in practice they usually mean 'community-oriented health care'. The initiative and the ownership of the programme remain with the NGO or the government institution that started the programme. One should consider statements like those of Francis Mburu that 'Government-executed community-based health care' is a contradiction in terms, and that the result is often a 'rhetoric implementation of PHC' (Mburu 1979). An examination of 52 CBHC programmes funded by USAID, all claiming that they promoted people's participation, showed that participation was mainly confined to implementation, and there was very little participation in decision-making and evaluation.

One of the main reasons that true CBHC has been difficult to implement has been that there is a large gap between the people initiating the process of change, who have their own theories and perceptions about what should be done, and the people in the community who are expected to respond with their own momentum. Such gaps may exist even where all the actors are from the same cultural background.

The development of CBHC challenges existing power structures. As Selina's text makes clear, people trained in western health care models are reluctant to give up the power that comes from the ownership of technologies and from their place in the institutional hierarchy. Real community participation implies that the professionals must transfer some of the decision-making power to the communities, which means they must give up some of their own power. They are called on to watch and listen, instead of simply bringing solutions. As Selina put it, 'Instead of going to teach, we go to learn.'

Redefining power structures is a process which always goes through several stages. It is often tough, involving conflicts between the community and those in charge of the programme, and also between community actors and the political structure, since redefining power also has a political dimension. At the level of organisations, there is often further conflict between people within the health services who have changed their attitudes and approaches in the process of developing community participation, and others who have not changed – and who may well be superior in the organisational hierarchy.

However, there are some models for community participation that have been successful in getting people together at community level to promote health. We are not attempting to make an exhaustive survey here, but we would like to mention a few organisations we know personally, and examine briefly the conditions that have helped them to be successful. Many of these programmes are carried out by small NGOs, which have a high level of grass-roots participation in the organisation as a whole. They function in different ways, but have in common a high level of local participation. For example in the West Bengal Voluntary Health Association, Calcutta, local groups hire health professionals on their own terms to supply health services, which enables them to 'own' their project. Families who are members pay regular financial contributions which enable the group to pay for regular health services and to fund other health-enhancing activities like improving water supplies and sanitation. Sustainability is often better assured when a nurse-midwife is chosen as the key health provider, but the people themselves often aspire to the more expensive – and often less appropriate – medical doctor.

Other models are found in Bangladesh. *Dushtha Shasthya Kendra* (DSK) is a large NGO based in Dhaka which has established a credit union to which smaller savings groups subscribe and share in the economic activities. The credit groups save part of their money for health care. In the north of Bangladesh a large NGO, Rajpur Dinajpur Rural Service (RDRS) works with credit groups whose members have access to a defined primary level health service package (the Essential Service Package) for its members, and provides referral services at a discount. The members have only a limited opportunity to determine the content of the service, but through the organised groups they can express their needs and concerns, and decide whether to take part or not. Another NGO, the Bangladesh Rural Advancement Committee, BRAC, has been active since 1972, with a variety of programmes aimed at 'sustainable self-reliance' (Lovell & Abed 1993). The aim is to empower people to manage their own health. An early activity in health was the development of a solution for Oral Rehydration Therapy (ORT) that could be prepared by village women from local ingredients, followed by a big education campaign to teach people how to use it. Educational campaigns also aim to make people more aware of the need for PHC services so that they bring pressure to bear on the government to supply them (Streefland & Chabot 1990).

Many community health programmes are based on local groups. For example, the Ghanaian Red Cross runs Mothers' Clubs, which Selina once visited for an exchange of experiences. In Jamkhed, India, there is a Comprehensive Rural Health Programme which has been working for 30 years. This programme, like that of the Care Groups, began with health provision and soon added a range of other activities to improve health and well-being. Because in this part of India women did not take part in public life, the activities began with farmer's clubs for men, which included health as well as agriculture in their programme. This was followed by the training of selected local women as village health workers, and then by the development of women's development associations, *Mahila Vikas Mandals* (Arole & Arole 1994, Jamkhed 2002).

In East Africa, an organisation that has many similarities to the Elim Care Group Movement is the CBHC programme of the Kakamega diocese in Western Kenya. The project was started by staff of the hospital in Nangina, near the Ugandan border, and supported by doctors from *Memisa* (the Dutch branch of Medicus Mundi). This was one of the first such projects, and was discussed in Alma Ata as an example of a project where involving the community had really altered the people's health status. As in Elim, one woman, Gertrude Lwanga, has played an important role. She trained at Nangina Hospital as a public health nurse, and then moved to the hospital at Mumias as PHC Co-ordinator. She extended the project to include two diocesan hospitals and their designated health areas, with a population of half a million.

The project in Kakamega started by training community health workers (CHW), but there is now a lot of emphasis on training the community's own resource persons (CORP). The aim is to enable them to identify and prioritise community problems, and to find solutions. The project helps communities to identify partners and networks that can help them to tackle their own problems. The term 'health problems' is considered to include any problem that threatens people or their environment. The project runs a variety of activities, including a number concerned with AIDS. One of these is called, 'Men and Traditions against AIDS', and aims at encouraging men to change their behaviour by educating the old men who are the policy makers and custodians of tradition.

A recent evaluation (CBHC 1997) showed that the programme had achieved some of its objectives, like reducing malnutrition in the area. The groups are still working along the lines of achieving predetermined health outputs, defined by the project management, but gradually more initiatives for planning and training are coming from the community itself. However, there are problems. As sometimes happened in the Care Group Project, conflicts between the CBHC team and the hospital management are a perennial problem, showing that there are still two different worlds. In addition, as it is a church project there are diocesan officials who also play a part. The needs of community empowerment do not fit well with the needs of the hospital management for ownership of the project, and with the financial obligations of the management to the donors. Another major problem is that the project is still perceived as belonging to the hospital, and CHWs feel that they should be paid for their work. They also complain that as volunteers they are not treated respectfully by hospital staff. During the evaluation, concern was often expressed about whether a project depending on volunteers could be sustainable. In Mumias, there is an emphasis on training administrative leaders and representatives of other sectors, to try to get broader support for the programme.

9. Conclusion: the Care Group Project as a model for CBHC

The discussion of our experience of the Care Group Project in this chapter has left us with more open questions than answers. Often, we only saw in retrospect how the problems arose, and we failed to address them at the time and find a good mechanism to solve them. Many of the problems were the result of the complexities of running a project that involved both the public health services and a voluntary organisation, but we remain convinced that if good co-operation and communication between the two sides can be developed, such collaboration can bring major advantages for both.

However, true Community Based Health Care requires the presence of a third actor – the community. If CBHC is to function and become sustainable, it demands the involvement of the members of the community – the ordinary citizens of villages and towns – not as passive recipients of the project's ideas but as active partners. As we discussed in the last section, there are only a few projects as yet in which this vision has been successfully put into practice, and shown results in terms of measurable improvements in health status, increased awareness about health, and the empowerment of previously marginalised people, especially women. The Elim Care Group Project is one of them, and the Kenyan project discussed above is another.

One thing that both these programmes, and many others, have in common is the leadership of an extremely strong person who was able to bridge the gap between modern concepts of health promotion and a culturally-determined traditional system. Such leaders share many characteristics. One is an enormously high level of frustration tolerance, that has enabled them to stick doggedly to the track they had decided to follow, despite being pushed around by the leadership of the health care institutions, and often misunderstood by the communities they worked with. To absorb abuse from health administrators, medical and nursing staff on the one side, and from those community leaders who mistrusted representatives from a different world on the other side, needs a special single-mindedness of thinking and purpose. It is women like Selina Maphorogo and Gertrude Lwanga who have made community-based health care systems – which can easily be designed at the conference table but are so difficult to implement at the level of the local community – into reality.

When the Elim Care Group Project began, all the people who initiated it and helped to lead and direct it were 'learning on the job' about how to run a community health project. Over the years, they acquired a lot of experience and a lot of insight into the process of developing projects together with a community. Although the Project – like every project and programme – grew up in a unique setting, many of these insights have a wider relevance. We hope that the story of the Care Group Movement, and Selina Maphorogo's memories of her 28 years of work as a Care Group Motivator, will help people who are planning and implementing similar projects to reach their goal more rapidly, and encounter fewer obstacles on the way.

Appendix

Bibliography

Glossary

Some practical instructions

Growing vegetables using the deep trench method [1]
Making and using a Wonder Box [2]
Making and using a Wood Stove [2]

[1] From Sutter E., Foster A. & Francis V. (1989) *Hanyane: a village struggles for eye health*. London: Macmillan.

[2] These pages are taken, with permission from the Care Group Project, from the special edition of the Care Group magazine *Care – Looking back and Looking Forward* produced to celebrate the 10th anniversary of the Project by Carel IJsselmuiden, Raymond de Swardt, Mokgadi Tlakula, Joseph Baloyi, Selina Maphorogo and other Motivators.

Bibliography

Books and documents referred to in the text

Arole M. & Arole R. (1994) *Jamkhed : a comprehensive rural health project.*
London: Macmillan

Ballard R.C., Sutter E.E. & Fotheringham P. (1978) *Trachoma in a Rural South African Community.* J. Trop. Med. Hyg. 27, 113-120

Boon, Mike (1996) *The African Way – the power of interactive leadership.* South Africa: Zebra Press, Struik Book Distributors

Chambers, Robert (1983) *Rural Development, putting the last first.* London: Longman

CBHC (1997) *Mid-Term Evaluation Report, CBHC Programmes, Mumias and Mukumu.* PHC/CBHC St Mary's Hospital, Mumias (P.O.Box 250, Mumias, Kenya) & PHC/CBHC St Elizabeth Hospital, Mukumu (P.O.Box 127, Kakamenga, Kenya)

Cohen J.M. & Uphoff N.T. (1980) *Participation's place in rural development: seeking clarity through specificity.* World Development 8, 213-235

Gyekye, Kwame (1995) *An essay on African philosophical thought: the Akan conceptual scheme.* Philadelphia: Temple University Press, pp.169 - 177

Hilton, Dave (1988) *Community-based or Community-oriented, the vital difference.* Contact (Christian Medical Commission, Geneva) 106, 1-13

Jamkhed (2002) *CRHP: Comprehensive Rural Health Project.* www.jamkhed.org

Lovell C. & Abed F.H. (1993) *Scaling-up in health: Two decades of Learning in Bangladesh.* In: Rohde J., Chatterjee M. & Morley D. (eds) (1993) *Reaching health for all.* Delhi: Oxford University Press

Macdonald John J. (1994) *Primary Health Care. Medicine in its place.* London: Earthscan Publications

Mbiti, John S. (1969) *African religions and philosophy.* London, Ibadan, Nairobi: Heinemann

Glossary

AEO
Agricultural Extension Officer

Cataract
Opacity of the crystalline lens of the eye, causing blindness.

CBHC
Community Based Health Care

Childhood blindness
The most common cause in Africa and East Asia is Vitamin A deficiency causing *xerophthalmia* (night blindness, and a dry eye followed by destruction of the cornea), usually coupled with malnutrition and measles. Eating green vegetables and/or yellow fruit daily would prevent the condition.

CHW
Community Health Worker

Civic Groups
Formerly these were ANC (African National Congress) activist groups, and suffered persecution. Since the change of Government, the groups consist of representatives of all community groups and structures, working together with the chief.

Clinic
In the South African health system, a clinic is a peripheral health point, staffed with a nurse and a nursing assistant, who can attend to minor ailments, run mother-and-child clinics, etc.

Deep Trench method of vegetable gardening
A method that allows vegetables to be grown in arid, poor-quality soils.
(See box on Valley Trust, page 77)

Donga
A gully caused by soil erosion.

Drought Relief Fund
A Government project to help people to create work for the poorest people in the communities. One activity was to start vegetable gardens, using the deep trench method.
(See also page 111)

Glaucoma
Increased pressure inside the eye which damages structures within the eye and leads to blindness, if not treated. It often goes untreated because it is painless.

Javel
A chlorine-containing bleaching fluid, commonly used in rural households.

Kwashiorkor
Protein/energy malnutrition. The child becomes swollen and apathetic, and suffers from skin lesions. The hair becomes discoloured and fluffy.

Leucaena tree
A quick-growing tree often recommended for firewood plantations etc. (See page 80)

Manani
Tsonga word for addressing women with respect: 'Mother, Madam, Mrs.'

Marasmus
Not enough food of all types, resulting in the skin-and-bone child with an enlarged abdomen.

Matric
Examination taken after 12 years' schooling, required for many training courses and for higher education.

Mavoni
Tsonga word for discharging eyes in a young child.

Mealie meal
Coarse maize meal, ground in a mill.

Mud stove
Home-built stove made of unburned mud bricks, designed to save fuel. (See illustration and building instructions: Appendix p. 268)

Mufundisi
Tsonga for pastor.

NGO
Non-Governmental Organisation

Nursing assistants or assistant nurses
The people who do the lowliest jobs in the nursing profession. They require education up to Standard 6 (8 school years).

N'wina
Tsonga for 'you' plural; the polite form for addressing an adult or respected person (traditionally, also for addressing a boy).

Oral rehydration fluid
A sugar/salt solution for the treatment of diarrhoea. The Care Group method: 1 teaspoon of salt and 8 teaspoons of sugar in 1 litre of previously boiled water. Treatment: with every stool, one 250 ml mug of solution given to the child with a spoon.

PHC
Primary Health Care

'Private teacher'
If there is a lack of qualified teachers, persons without a teacher's training can be employed, receiving a lower salary, but paid by the state.

Pterygium
A triangular thickening of the nasal part of the conjunctiva, encroaching on the cornea. In Africa the overgrowth of the cornea may cause visual impairment.

Road-to-Health Chart
A widely-used chart for Child Health clinics in developing countries, used to monitor the child's growth (weight for age).

Rondavel
A one-roomed house with a conical grass roof.

Sangoma
Tsonga for herbalist or traditional healer. Most of them also use some magic.

Shinyeku
Tsonga word for in-turning eye lashes with or without blindness. Also used to describe a careless, poor woman.

Soft porridge
Soft maize meal porridge.

Standard 6
The 8th school year at the end of which a certificate is issued after examination. It is the minimum required for many jobs like nursing assistant.

Sunbeams
Junior branch of the 'Wayfarers' (the Girl Guide organisation for Black South Africans).

Tindluwa
Tsonga name for ground-beans. These are a species of groundnut, and grow with the pods underground.

Tiribi
The Care Groups' name for oral rehydration fluid.

Throwing bones
Traditional healers and diviners use a collection of small bones which they throw onto a mat when counselling a client. From the resulting pattern of the bones the healer or diviner can read the required treatment, the client's future – or, in case of misfortune or a disaster, the person guilty of inflicting the curse.

Trachoma
A preventable eye disease that occurs predominantly in arid areas in the southern hemisphere, caused by the bacterium *Chlamydia trachomatis* (See box on page 32)

VIP toilet
Ventilated Improved Pit toilet. The special construction of these toilets reduces smells and flies.

Vitamin A deficiency
See 'Childhood blindness'.

Vuswa
Tsonga and Venda word for a stiff maize meal porridge produced from maize pounded by hand.

Wayfarers
Name for the (Black) South African Girl Guides, to separate them from the 'real' (White) Girl Guides. Members of the junior branch were called 'Sunbeams'.

Wena
Tsonga for 'you' singular; familiar form used for addressing a child or a near friend.

Wonder box
A box fitted with two insulating cushions, used to save fuel. If food is brought to the boil and the pot is then placed between the cushions, it will go on cooking slowly for some hours. (See page 79. Illustration and sewing instructions: Appendix p. 266)

Xerophthalmia
See under 'Childhood blindness'.

Zionist church
The 'Zion Christian Church' was founded at the end of the 19th century by its bishop Engenase Lekganyane. It broke away from the Lutheran Church, because people felt they were not treated as equals by the white missionaries. It is one of the largest of the many independent, partly syncretistic churches in South Africa, and very popular in the Northern Province.

Some practical instructions

HOW TO MAKE A TRENCH FOR VEGETABLE GROWING

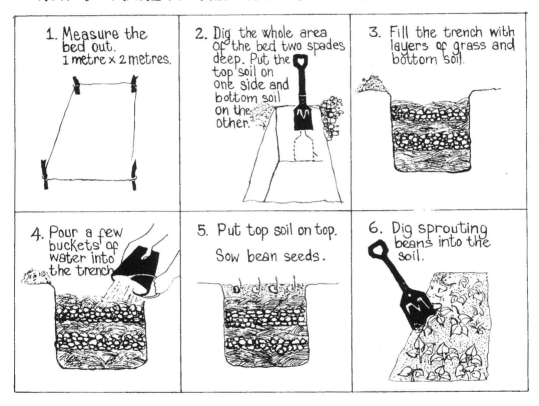

1. Measure the bed out. 1 metre × 2 metres.

2. Dig the whole area of the bed two spades deep. Put the top soil on one side and bottom soil on the other.

3. Fill the trench with layers of grass and bottom soil.

4. Pour a few buckets of water into the trench.

5. Put top soil on top. Sow bean seeds.

6. Dig sprouting beans into the soil.

WHAT TO USE

You can use any cloth material. You can buy COTTON or use an old mealie meal bag.

(Don't use plastic or nylon).

Cut **4** pieces to make the COVER

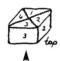

Sew the pieces together as in these drawings

Cut **4** pieces to make the BASE into which you can put the pot

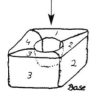

THE WONDER BOX

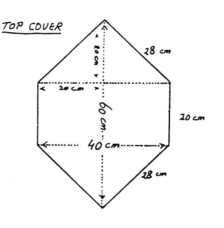

TOP COVER

28 cm
10 cm
20 cm
60 cm
20 cm
40 cm
28 cm

BASE

20 cm
28 cm
40 cm
20 cm
80 cm
20 cm
30 cm
10 cm
12 cm
12 cm
12 cm
12 cm
12 cm
17 cm

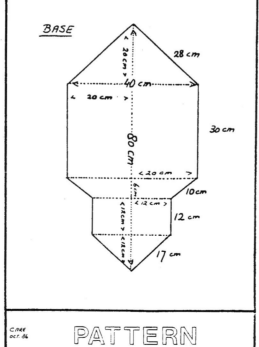

CARE
oct. 86

PATTERN

THE FILLING

You can use any materials that keep the heat to fill up your wonder box:
- polystyrene pieces or granules
- peanut shells
- old newspaper (make small balls)
- grass
- feathers

DON'T FILL TOO MUCH otherwise the pot does not fit well

KEEP IT NICE

Your wonder box will last a long time. Protect it by putting it in a wooden box or a carton, or even in a big clay pot!

WHO CAN USE IT?

- you
- your family
- your neighbours
- all the other people in the village

TELL THEM!

WHY SHOULD YOU USE A WONDER BOX ????

1. It can save a lot of wood or other fuel : sometimes as much as **half** your normal use !

2. You can leave it UNATTENDED and do other things.

3. The food can not burn or boil over !

4. It is SAFE · there is no fire !!

5. You can prepare food in the morning and have a nice hot meal when you come back in the afternoon. (or the children coming back from school can eat while the mother works)

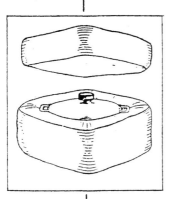

Cook smart: use the WONDER BOX

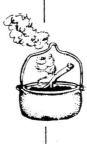

HOW SHOULD YOU USE THE WONDER BOX ?????

1. Put water and food in the cooking pot.

2. Bring the pot to the boil on a fire or (even better) on your wood-stove.

3. Let it boil for a short time (= 5 minutes).

4. Take the pot from the fire and put it in the wonder box.
   Make sure that the cushions of the wonder box cover the pot on all sides.

5. EAT when you and your food are ready :

   for example : – rice : $\frac{1}{2}$ hour
   – mealie meal : 1 hour
   – beans : 3 hours
   – meat (stew) : 5-6 hours

USE A WOOD-STOVE!

•• 2 AND 3 POT MODELS ••

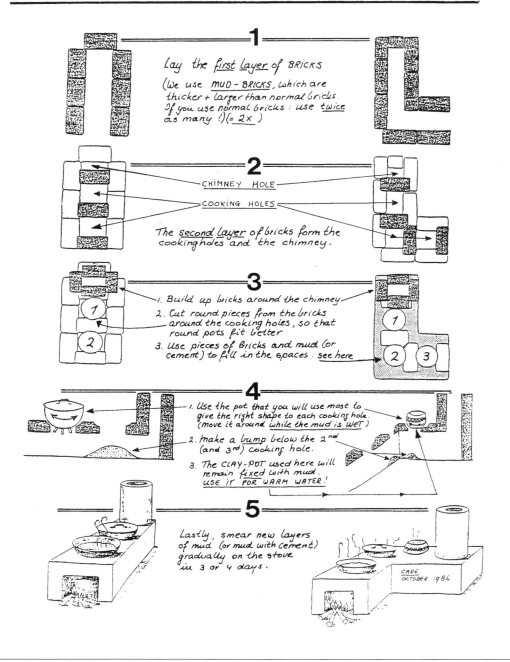

1

Lay the _first layer_ of BRICKS

(We use _MUD - BRICKS_, which are thicker + larger than normal bricks. If you use normal bricks : use _twice_ as many !)(= _2x_)

2

CHIMNEY HOLE

COOKING HOLES

The _second layer_ of bricks form the cookingholes and the chimney.

3

1. Build up bricks around the chimney.
2. Cut round pieces from the bricks around the cooking holes, so that round pots fit better
3. Use pieces of bricks and mud (or cement) to fill in the spaces : _see here_

4

1. Use the pot that you will use most to give the right shape to each cooking hole. (move it around _while the mud is WET_)
2. make a _bump_ below the 2nd (and 3rd) cooking hole.
3. The CLAY-POT used here will remain _fixed_ with mud. _USE IT FOR WARM WATER!_

5

Lastly, smear new layers of mud (or mud with cement) gradually on the stove in 3 or 4 days.

CARE
OCTOBER 1986

THE REASONS FOR COOKING ON A WOOD-STOVE
(instead of cooking on an open fire)

1. It can save a lot of wood ! A mother now has to fetch only half the wood that she normally has to fetch, and so, she has more time for her children. *It also preserves our trees!*

2. Your fire place is now SAFE for children, older people and people suffering from epilepsy.

3. The fire can remain UNATTENDED for a whole day !

4. You can have HOT WATER during the whole day: this will improve hygiene and will make your time spent on cooking shorter.

5. The kitchen will remain a bit warm during the night : it will be very comfortable in winter.

6

You can still improve your stove in 3 ways, as follows :

1. Before building the stove, make a foundation of 3-5 bricks high ⇒ then you can do your cooking standing !

2. Connect the chimney to a hole in the wall of your kitchen ⇒ then you can cook without smoke !

3. If you make a foundation, you can use it also to make an oven ! ⇒ to bake bread and cakes.
   → Just leave a big hole below and to the side of the fire-place. You can close off the oven by using a piece of iron.

4. Slide in a metal plate in the opening : by closing it your fire will burn less fast and this saves even more wood.

USE 2 EMPTY TINS WITH THE BOTTOM CUT OUT TO MAKE THE CHIMNEY-PIPE

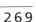